****

Sanctity of Life
Pitted Against
Quality of Life

****

Ethical Medical Decisions at the Bedside
With and For
the
Sole Good of the Patient

****

Robert Henry Crumby

Copyright © 2012 Robert H. Crumby
All rights reserved.
ISBN: 1479165263
ISBN-13: 978-1479165261

Book Cover by Joey Hayes, Pivotal Creative Design.
Unless otherwise indicated, the Scripture quotations contained herein are from the New Revised Standard Version Bible (NRSV), copyright 1989, Division of Christian Education of the National Council of the Churches of Christ in the United States of America. All rights reserved.
The King James Version will be cited KJV.

In loving memory

of

Taylor Coleman, Mary McMillan Moore, Ruth Stanley and Lorene Sharp White

With whose lives and deaths the author was personally familiar and involved. Their intermittent and end-of-life stories appear in this book and are used with permission of the respective families, along with more public narratives.

Dedicated to

Our Grandchildren

Luke   Caleb   Hannah   Molly   Franklin   Keaton

CONTENTS

Prologue   Through the Clinical Netherworld

Part One   1

I	Moral Evaluation in the Clinical Ethos	2
II	Living Courageously with Disease—Injury—Impairment (Helen Keller, Mary Moore, Lorene Sharp White)	15
III	Overcoming the Netherworld: Claiming a Good Death(Ruth Stanley)	37
IV	Playing God	47
V	Culture of Denial	55
VI	Technological Delusions	63
VII	Quality of Life Pitted against Sanctity of Life	74

Part Two   86

VIII	Whole-Brain Death (Taylor Coleman)	88
IX	Neocortical Disaster—Persistent Vegetative State (Karen Ann Quinlan)	98
X	PVS (Continuation) (Nancy Cruzan, Terri Schiavo, Paul Brophy)	118
XI	Implications for Denial of Justice at the End of Life	138
	Diagram of Brain	148

Part Three   **150**

XII   Locked-in Syndrome (John Doe I)   151
Basilar Artery Bifurcation Aneurism
(John Doe II)
Locked-in Syndrome (Jean Dominique Bauby)

XIII   Amyotrophic Lateral Sclerosis
(Lou Gehrig, Jane Doe, and Nancy Gamble)   169

Epilogue   180

Appendix: Acknowledgments, Notes,
And Helping Agencies   181

Profound Thanks Are Extended
to
Bavarian Professor Georg Hermann Dellbrugge
Professor John Lachs
Professor Daniel Maguire
Professor, Physician, Lawyer Bruce D. White
Professor Richard Zaner

Prologue

Through the Clinical Netherworld

If life is a journey, as the poets suggest, sooner or later that pilgrimage takes one through the *netherworld.* The "clinical" netherworld is an extreme low point that can be a living hell for those who suddenly find themselves and their loved ones trying to understand the complex health-care and moral issues confronting them at some point in their lives or at life's end.

The purpose of this book is to address the lay public and those patients and their spiritual, psycho-social, medical, and nursing advisors who may have only rudimentary knowledge of the ethics and morality of clinical procedures intermittently and at the end of life. It is intended to be a pastoral discourse, a primer to be read by laypersons or to be used by pastors and other health-care professionals in conversations or teaching settings with their parishioners or clients.

The expanded process in presenting these case studies includes not only the relevant medical and ethical details but also the intimate spiritual, psycho-social, fiscal, and legal data encompassing the patient and the family. A particular focus is upon the harsh rigors faced by the individual patients, but subsequently on the painful anguish of the families as well—along with the compassionate involvement of other caregivers in the starkness of the settings where critically ill persons are observed and treated in the immediacy of the moment at the netherworld bedside.

Initial argument is made that the first goals of medicine are to affirm the sacredness of human life and, in the clinical ethos, to relieve pain and discomfort along with diagnosing and curing disease. In due course, however, every sparrow falls to the ground. Human life, though of greatest natural value, is not infinite. Commensurately, many persons die too soon and their families and friends are often not prepared to let them go. Thousands of other human beings are sustained in horribly debilitated, brain-damaged, and financially costly conditions for indeterminable periods of time, in states worse than death. This book is not about suicide, mercy killing, or assisted suicide. It is an effort to enable patients, families, pastors, lawyers, physicians, and nurses, negotiating within the clinical encounter, to make reasonable and humane decisions on the withholding and withdrawal of non-beneficial and expensive treatment—or, when medically indicated, to effect palliative care until natural death occurs. Although not its central theme, this work brings full circle the vital connection between brain death and the critically important issues of body part transplantation and puts a human face on the distressful recipients who plaintively wait in the shadows.

Part One

Using the "clinical ethos" as a framing statement for ethical procedure and as a point of departure, our journey through the clinical netherworld will continue in this initial section with the short and long-term physically and mentally conflicted and their caregivers. Wandering much of their lives in and out of grim clinical environments, such persons often display unusual gifts of spirit in the face of disease, injury, and impairment, which encumber humankind, as well as the flight and subsequent fall of the sparrow. Multimillions of Americans struggle emotionally, mentally, and physically every day, individuals for whom the doors of hope remain open. These are the medically challenged who are courageously striving to overcome maladies for which health-care intervention may yet have perceivable and measurable benefit.

Beginning with a definitive respect for values in the natural order and the sanctity of human life, we lift up the goals of medicine, articulated by Canadian-born physician William Osler, widely acclaimed as the father of modern medicine—goals that reach out to these hopeful individuals: "To prevent disease, to relieve suffering, and to heal the sick—this is our work."[1] A word of mitigation is presented as worthy of consideration, that along with our initial dedication to the task of sensitive and aggressive health care delivery, we acknowledge the limits of medicine and human life, resisting society's penchant for denial of death. Clinical encounters may become issues of sanctity of life pitted against quality of life, calling for heart-rending decisions in the midst of ethical dilemmas.

Chapter I

Moral Evaluation in the Clinical Ethos

Compassionate professionals, ethically evaluating, discussing, and implementing treatment options at the bedside with a patient or surrogate, are "doing" clinical ethics. Reference is made to doing ethics since those involved are actively negotiating a wide range of values to guide choices, which lead to their respective and collective decisions. At the close of the nineteenth century, Professor of Philosophy John S. McKenzie, at the University of South Wales developed for his students a manual of *ethics*, which he introduced as "The Science of the Ideal in Conduct." He declares at the outset:

> The term 'ethics' stems from the Greek words *athos* meaning character and *ethos* meaning custom or habit. Similarly, the term 'moral philosophy,' which means the same thing as ethics, is derived from the Latin *mores,* meaning habits or customs. . . .The term 'right' is derived from the *Latin rectus*, meaning 'straight' or 'according to rule.' The term 'good' is connected to the German *gut,* and contains the same root as the Greek *agathos.* A thing is said to be good when it is valuable to some end.[1]

The "clinic" is the place where sick or injured persons are observed and treated for the sole *good* of the patient. It is endemic to the institutional hospital, the nursing facility, the private home, the hospice, the Mobile Army Surgical Hospital (MASH), the shipboard infirmary, or any other comparable setting. To travel through the clinical netherworld is a gut-wrenching, soul-searching, and often heart-breaking encounter of mental and spiritual highs and lows. Encapsulated, there is often no more surreal a place on Earth for patients, families, and friends than this uncharted territory. Ironically, modern technology presents in these settings as both a blessing and a curse. In concert with nature's laws, professional caregivers daily stretch the parameters of life and effect recoveries and ultimate cures that are miraculous. But the natural limitations are there too, creating complex ethical dilemmas—conflicts in faith and practice, in values and decisions, in acceptance and denial—when quality of life presents itself as conditional.

Affixing sacredness and value to the life of a person, as well as to a person's conduct and relationship with others, is the function of ethics and morality, processes that appear in both secular and religious history. Much of the data to follow is supportive of that argument. That there is eternal and universal value in each person's life and each person's death is embodied in the thoughts and writings of Catholic moral philosopher/professor Daniel Maguire. I suggest that descriptive materials from his most recent book constitute a vital starting point for evaluating the clinical ethos specifically, as well as for framing a social and political ethics in general. Dr. Maguire writes:

> The terms *moral, sacred, the sanctity of life* are meaningful across cultures . . . the concept of the sanctity of life undergirds all the laws of all peoples . . . the **foundational moral experience** is the experience of the value of persons and their earthly home in this universe. This profound value experience is the distinctively human and humanizing experience and the gateway to personhood.[2]

There is no process in our communal life where a philosophy of medical diagnosis/prognosis, ethical procedure, and sanctity of life is more important than health-care decision making in clinical settings. There is no professional-client relationship more indefatigably value laden than the physician/patient encounter where the patient's health and life are at stake. Such recognition evokes physician Eric Cassell's belief that, "medicine is inherently a moral profession—or a moral technical profession, if you wish . . . moral because it has directly to do with the welfare and good of others."[3] It enhances physician Edmund Pelligrino's affirmation that medicine is "The most humane of sciences, the most empiric of arts, and the most scientific of humanities."[4]

Our search for foundational principles on the sanctity of life and medical ethics takes us to ancient times by way of the Hebrew tradition, to the golden age of Israel in tenth century BC onward. It was from this period that the poetic hymns in worship and the fervent passion of the prophets in the public square mingled with Hebrew law, the Torah, passing down through the Psalter, Talmud, and Mishnah to become the moral fabric of succeeding generations. There was no doubt in the Hebrew mind that in the economy of God human life was a value of the first order, surpassed by no other value, as affirmed in a psalm attributable to King David, a musician and hymnist whom ancient texts described as the "sweet psalmist of Israel:"[5]

> O Lord, our Sovereign,
> how majestic is your name in all the earth! . . .
> When I look at your heavens, the work of your fingers,
> the moon and the stars, that you have established;
> what are human beings that you are mindful of them,
> mortals that you care for them?
> Yet you have made them a little lower than God,
> and crowned them with glory and honor.
> You have given them dominion over the works of your hands;
> you have put all things under their feet.[6]

In a book on medical ethics, Georgetown Professor Robert Veatch writes with emphasis on the value of human life as found in the history of Jewish medical ethics and presents data that has both ancient and modern relevance: "While many wrongly interpret the central core of the Hippocratic tradition as committing the physician to preserve life, this is a central precept of the Jewish medical ethic. Jews, whether they be physicians or laypersons, are the original advocates of the right to life at almost any cost."[7]

Nonetheless, I will argue that such facts do not diminish the ancient Greek patterns of melding ethics and morality with medical practice at an elementary level. Widespread medical traditions point to a period in secular history on both sides of the year 400 BC, to the physician Hippocrates who, according to Alexandrian accounts, was born in 460 BC.[8] This biographical note refers to an era in which,

"The figure of legendary Father of Medicine soon replaced the historical Hippocrates." The terms *legendary* and *historical* relate to the fact that: "Although there is no evidence from his own time that he left any writings, within a century medical works were being attributed to Hippocrates, especially those emanating from the famous medical school of Cos."[9]

Certainly the most familiar of the attributions related to this ancient physician is the Hippocratic Oath, which bore his name through the historical development of medical practice from ancient eras into modern and contemporary times. At the very least, these principles contain vital elements of duty and obligation, and constitute a moral posture beyond ordinary communal activities and professional conduct. Physician Edmund Pelligrino writes: "The central and most admirable feature of the oath is the respect it inculcates for the patient. In the oath, the doctor is pledged always to help the patient and keep him from harm."[10]

Flowing initially from the secular Hippocratic tradition are two significant moral principles, historically and universally related to medical ethics, the principles of non-maleficence and beneficence. The first rule of medical professional conduct, non-maleficence, springs from the Latin injunctive phrase *primum non necere*, "first do no harm." Beneficence, the second, correlatively, is the "striving for good" in behalf of the patient. These maxims are the linchpins that held together the moral duty of the clinical practitioner and constituted an ethical concern for the life of the person in ancient Greece.

A portion of the Hippocratic Oath itself reflects the essence of these two principles, with the positive one first and the prohibitive one second: "I will follow that system of regimen which, according to my ability and judgment, I consider for the benefit of my patients, and abstain from whatever is deleterious and mischievous."[11] In my view, these two maxims initiated a moral framework for the practice of medicine within an age of ancient paganism and paved the way for greater ethical pluralism in the centuries to come.

As for the Christian faith, in addition to the Jewish beliefs, both Roman Catholic and Protestant bioethical traditions show themselves to be manifestations of the "foundational moral experience" espoused earlier by Professor Maguire, that is, "the value of persons and their earthly home in this universe." An article appearing in the Canadian Medical Association Journal is a worthy representation of the Roman Catholic position on the value of human life. It is consistent with Maguire's aforementioned premise:

> There is a long tradition of bioethical reasoning within the Roman Catholic Faith, a tradition that extends from Augustine's writings on suicide in the early Middle Ages to recent papal teachings on euthanasia and reproductive technologies. . . . Fundamental to Catholic bioethics is a belief in the sanctity of life: the value of a human life, as a creation of God and a gift in trust, is beyond human evaluation and authority.[12]

Mingling with the twenty-eight hundred years of Judeo-Christian-Catholic tradition, is the Protestant counterpoise development under the dynamic leadership of the twin towers, the excommunicated German priest Martin Luther and the French/Swiss lawyer/theologian John Calvin in the sixteenth century AD. Through them and others, Protestantism likewise celebrates the critical importance of affirming a doctrine of the sacredness of human life and care for the dying. Evidence of this claim is manifest in the twentieth-century neo-orthodoxy of Swiss theologian Karl Barth and the reaffirmation of earlier reformed theological principles following a period of nineteenth-century liberalism. In his *Church Dogmatics,* Barth writes:

> As God the Creator calls man to himself and turns him to his fellow-man. He orders him to honour his own life and that of every other man as a loan and to secure it against all caprice, in order that it may be used in this service and in preparation for this service.[13]
> What matters is that everyone should treat his existence and that of every other human being with respect. For it belongs to God. It is His loan and blessing.[14]
> We cannot and must not seriously tire of life. For it is always an offer waiting for man's will, determination

and readiness for action. And it is to be noted that this is real respect for life.[15]

In 1981 the Presbyterian Church U.S., an entity within the protestant reformed tradition, approved a report of its Committee on Theology and Culture: "The Nature and Value of Human Life." In part, this theological statement with medical implications reflects the revelatory respect for life in the commandments given to the Jews and Christians. Secondly, there are provisos remarkably similar to the secular ones of those in the school of Hippocrates (non-maleficence and beneficence):

> The value of human life is based upon God's creation, preservation, and redemption of it. . . . Explicit scriptural expression of this respect for life is found in the commandment to do no unjustifiable killing. . . . The reformed tradition has discerned several elements in this command. The first is the obligation to avoid doing harm. A second is the obligation to protect and preserve life by doing that which sustains it.[16]

Joining non-maleficence and beneficence, two additional moral maxims have emerged from ancient times and apply to the valuing of life and to medical ethics decision making, the principles of autonomy and justice. The first one, *autonomy*, is a derivative of two Greek words *auto* (self) and *nomos* (law), which conjoined essentially reflect the principle of self-determination. When Thomas Jefferson affirmed in the United States Declaration of Independence the natural law of self evidence "that all men are created equal and that they are endowed by their Creator with certain unalienable rights . . . Life, Liberty, and the Pursuit of Happiness,"[17] he profoundly framed the principle of autonomy for the burgeoning young nation. In other words, as a living person of value, the autonomous individual should have the unfettered right to participate in the determination of his/her own destiny, especially pertinent to twenty-first-century health-care issues.

The overarching issue here is liberty—freedom to choose and to act—freedom for all, freedom for each. It must be noted that the principles of autonomy and justice here are conditioned by the harsh reality of history. The 1776 declaration of the "unfettered" right of citizens to participate in the franchise of liberty and justice for all was denied American Indians, African Americans, and all women in matters of political, economic, and social justice over many decades of American history. Thus, the implications for the "denial" of justice are matters of critical import. Such is argued in chapter XI of this book under the rubric of "delay" of justice as being tantamount to denial of justice in all matters, including health care delivery.

Be that as it may, such a concept of individual liberty was promulgated approximately 575 years earlier than 1776, at the broad plain of Runnymede, twenty-one miles west of London on the banks of the Thames and two miles from Windsor Castle. At that place on June 15, 1215, accompanied by legions of their armies, English barons presented a similar claim to England's King John and forced precepts written on parchment to be signed by the monarch on the spot (Magna Charta)–revised just a few years henceforth to become part of England's common law, and to impact centuries later the Declaration of Independence and the Constitution of the United States. The remarkable sixty-third and final precept, agreed to by absolute ruler King John, states in part: "Wherefore we will and firmly command . . . that the men in our kingdom shall have and hold all the aforesaid liberties, rights and concessions, well and peacefully, freely and quietly, fully and completely, for themselves and their heirs, in all things and places, forever as before said."[18]

Immanuel Kant in 1785, a professor at the University of Konigsburg in East Prussia, published materials that included forceful concepts of autonomy. He is considered to be one who has made a monumental contribution to the concept of what it means to be free and unrestrained in formulating moral, political, and social decisions. Kant's observations add huge impetus, I would argue, when applied to moral medical decisions and ethical procedures in the health-care setting: "Laws arise from the will, viewed generally as practical wisdom; maxims spring from the activity of the will in the process of choice. The latter in man is what constitutes free will. . . . It is, therefore, only the act of *choice* in the voluntary process that can be called *free.*"[19]

Allen D. Verhey, Ph.D., makes the case, from a religious perspective, that Protestant Christian theologians also have important perspectives to share on the issue of patient autonomy. He cites the importance of freedom and liberty when it comes to religious expression and activity: "One of the things Protestantism was from the very beginning . . . was freedom." Then, referring to Luther, he states later, "Protestants remain *for freedom*—also in medical ethics."[20] And, further along, Verhey reflects on the fact that philosophy has likewise made significant contributions to the issues of freedom and autonomy. He thus captures the essence of Kantian autonomy, which asserts, "The moral law could only be imposed on *one's self* and only through one's moral reasoning. The moral agent—to be a moral agent—had to choose and act in accordance with rational principles."[21] Essentially this argues for the principle, stated earlier, that not only must a person have the freedom to make ethical decisions but also must embrace a sense of duty or obligation along with the moral resolve to act.

As we shall see in subsequent chapters, the rights to autonomy and self-determination formulate themselves within the changing physician-patient relationship, from one of paternalism on the physician's part, to one of negotiation with the patient on decision-making matters within the clinical encounter. Conditionally, this claims for the patient the right to autonomy, the right to privacy, the right to be informed, the right to give consent or to refuse treatment, and ultimately the right to die. At the same it recognizes the autonomic rights of the physician along with institutional autonomy as well as the interface with communal values and laws. It also encourages patient surrogates to be more resolute in fostering advance directives of the patient when that individual has lost decision-making capacity, along with offering the right to act in the patient's best interests when the wishes of the patient are unknown.

Thomas Jefferson, in the "Declaration of Independence," affirms that "all men," not just one, are created equal, affirming that there are other individuals out there with whom the blessings of freedom and autonomy must be shared. That raises the question of "justice," the fourth principle which universally has been applied to issues presented by medical ethics. Not only to expect fair and equitable treatment for oneself, but to acknowledge the outward nature of justice, the recognition that every human being is a social being and exists in relationships without which no one can thrive, much less be born. In life, these relationships may be pitted against one another or find the common ground of mutuality, which is the essence of justice, widely diffused.

Again we turn to ancient Israel for examples of the heroic efforts of the solitary few who have railed against the greed and injustices perpetrated by those with power and influence throughout the early history of societies. Amos and Micah were prophetic eighth century BC voices calling for just reform in the midst of a theocratic culture, which had all but lost any sense of social and political fairness among its people. Amos emphatically castigates his countrymen for having broken their contract with God to be inclusive and morally circumspect: "you trample on the poor / and take from them levies of grain. . . . But let justice roll down like waters, / and righteousness like an ever flowing stream."[22]

The Hebrew word for righteousness, a word indicating virtuous acts toward others, was used interchangeably with and often in the place of the word justice. Micah was cogent and eloquent in his summarized formula for social reform: "He has told you, O mortal, what is good; / and what does the LORD require of you, / but to do justice, and to love kindness, / and to walk humbly with your God."[23] His terse enjoinder covered all of the law as well as the sum total of the proclamation of the prophets.

Seven hundred eighty-one miles across the Mediterranean and Aegean Seas, west-northwest of Israel, lay Athens-Attica of the fifth century BC, historically positioned between the Persian and Peloponnesian wars. It was, 445-431 BC, the age of the great statesman Pericles and others of his peers—poets, artists, politicians, and philosophers. They were attempting to craft for secular Athens what the eighth-century prophets were unable to do in theocratic Israel, to bring about egalitarian reform that would give the rank and file citizenry a fair share in the political, economic, and social life of the city/state (as indicated earlier, the issue of the actual delivery of justice to all, will be mitigated later in chapter 11). Athens, at this juncture however, was a noble experiment in the blending of autonomy and justice, as historian P.V.N. Myers notes:

> The people were at this period the source and fountain of all power. Every matter which concerned Athens and her empire was discussed by the popular assembly. Never before in the history of the world

had people enjoyed such unrestricted political liberty as did the citizens of Athens at this time, and never before were any people, through so intimate a knowledge of public affairs, so well fitted to take part in the administration of the government.[24]

Though a gifted orator, as much so or greater than Amos and Micah, Pericles sought to accomplish the administration of justice through a process of participatory democracy unique in history, differing in kind from the representative democracy centuries later in the United States. According to Professor P.V. N. Myers, "He ruled, as Plutarch says, by the art of persuasion."[25] Thus, we can conclude that Pericles was not in the strictly political sense a ruler but rather an enabler, as Myers goes on to observe: "It was a fixed idea of Pericles that in a democracy there should be not only an equal distribution of political rights among all classes, but also an equalization of the means and opportunities of exercising these rights, together with an equal participation by all in the social and intellectual enjoyments."[26]

Justice, standing alone in the clinical health-care situation is not enough, however, to deliver comprehensive moral decisions, nor is autonomy. Attempts are made to superimpose, individually or collectivity, the principles of non-maleficence, beneficence, autonomy, and justice, along with an assortment of other rules of conduct and ethical decision making, onto specific clinical cases. Such applications, devoid of a contextual framework of physician/patient negotiation and shared values, have appeared to be painfully inadequate. These endeavors, called "formative" or "applied" ethics, are found lacking as well in the onslaught of new technologies, new procedures, and remarkably effective new medicines. "The terms *value* and *purpose*" observes physician Edmund Pelligrino, "are beginning to appear for the first time as respectable subjects for clinical inquiry."[27]

Thus, Pelligrino offers a necessary caveat when evaluating the importance of the Hippocratic tradition for the clinical practice of medicine in the twenty-first century. Though of continuing importance in establishing a perspective on duty and the respect for the patient, the principles of non-maleficence and beneficence are lacking when formulating a foundation for complex medical ethics decision making in the post-modern clinical setting. "In a simpler world," says Pelligrino, "that ethic long sufficed to guide the physician in his service to the community. Today, the intersection of medicine with contemporary science, technology, social organization, and changed human values has revealed significant missing dimensions in the ancient ethic."[28]

Moral and ethical values, like virtues, must be initiated in order to be validated. The virtuous individual is morally abstract if that individual does not *act* virtuously. This is precisely why we speak of *doing* ethics. English moralist John S. Mackenzie in the late nineteenth century states forthrightly: "Virtue exists only in activity . . . goodness is not a capacity or potentiality but an activity. . . . The essence of virtue lies in the will."[29] Immanuel Kant wrote earlier, near the end of the eighteenth century, "Virtue signifies a moral strength of will . . . . Virtue then is the moral strength of a man's *will* in his obedience to *duty*"[30] Such moral incentive and activity is what contemporary poet Marguerite Wilkinson plaintively confesses that she lacks: "For I am haunted night and day, by all the deeds I have not done; O un-attempted loveliness! O costly valor never won!"[31]

Moral choice, even within life's most ordinary functions, is a process that presents to each of us every moment of our conscious existence and is especially vital in health-care decision making. Sociologist R.M. MacIver stated, "To live is to act, to act is to choose, and to choose is to evaluate."[32] In other words, if one is alive, choice is a virtual necessity and evaluation is an essential part of it. When a person is asleep, or in a coma, obviously there is no capacity for choosing. But, when a person awakens from sleep or a coma, sentient life mandates that decisions be made, unless that individual wants to spend the rest of his life in bed, or is enjoined by illness to do so. Under normal circumstances, an in-bed individual is aroused, perhaps stretches, rubs his eyes to remove the cobwebs, and maybe even lies there for a period, assessing the requirements of the day.

Then, MacIver's rubric for conduct comes into play. Some form of action takes place, and for that to happen choices are made, evaluation having preceded the subsequent decision to act. Does the person not feel well—needs or values more sleep—or does the individual respond to the reality that a busy schedule is calling for an early departure from home? Affixing value to one's life and conduct ordinarily propels the individual out of bed in response to the demands or responsibilities that have been accepted by that person at that point in time. Irresponsibility or illness may restrict the actions and commit the individual to another course.

"At any rate," stated Aristotle, "choice involves a rational principle and thought. Even the name seems to suggest that it is what is chosen before other things."[33] "Therefore," he says, "virtue also is in our power, and so too vice."[34] As we are confronted by the complexities of health-care decisions in a technologically driven society, values, or the lack of them, play an increasingly determinative role. The responsibility to choose is immanently present! "Moral issues," writes Richard Zaner, "are presented solely within the contexts of their actual occurence."[35]

Since valued human life and health are at stake, medical decisions made within the clinical ethos necessarily move us beyond the commonplace, often beyond one's own bedroom or comfort zone, invariably to confront more emotion-charged and complex issues in the clinical setting. Dr. Pelligrino shares a succinct observation, "But any attempt to define the virtuous physician or a virtue-based ethic for medicine must offer some definition of the good of the patient.... The patient's good is the end of medicine."[36] Moral choices in such an extended environment are compounded by the very nature of the setting, where strangers suddenly appear at one's bedside—where patient's minds and bodies are comprehensively explored in what Richard Zaner has also succinctly described as "Ethics and the Clinical Encounter."[37] A critical notation by Dr. Zaner is an apt conclusion to our moral evaluation of the clinical ethos. His statement on the necessary interconnections involved in the process of medical decision making concurs with the observations of Pelligrino and is a strategically important disclosure:

> The moral foundations of clinical medicine and of the experience of illness, not surprisingly, turn out to be profoundly interrelated and mutually determining. The therapeutic dyad of trust and care has its basis, on the one hand, in the 'moral chance' of illness and in the scientifically and linguistically informed clinical act of affiliative feeling, on the other. Because of the uniqueness of this relationship and the conversations and actions by which it is carried out as a process, it is an essentially moral relationship showing all the

characteristics of being fundamental to moral life. On the one side, the vulnerability and *appeal* of the ill person; on the other, the *response* from the would-be healer. Their relationship, deeply textured in our times by complex forms of social norms and institutions, complicated by strangers engaging in multiple forms of intimacy, is an essentially tenuous, unequal, and asymmetrical one, the very fact of which constitutes a complex and altogether special set of occasions for awakening our sense of morality in its core form.[38]

Thus, health care delivery within the clinical ethos is an unusually careful, complex, human procedure but, admittedly, is not error free. Physicians, nurses, technicians, ethics enablers, and administrative staff, however, are duty bound by their professional and institutional core values to deliver treatment and care which are reflective of the fiduciary, though asymmetric, relationship existing between them and their patients. William Osler's goals for medicine should be the *minimal* goals of all health-care procedure unless the burdens of treatment outweigh the benefits of treatment—or until death has rendered its final insult to a person's physical existence after long and courageous battles with disease—or has traumatically presented itself in manifestations of suddenness.

Chapter II

Living Courageously with Chronic Disease—Injury—Impairment

No one in this life has perfect health in body, mind, or spirit; it is a matter of degree. A sign in Nashville Summit Medical Center cardiac rehab offers this sober reminder: "Having good health simply means you're dying at the slowest possible rate."[1] There are levels of health moving upward to the good, better, or the best possible in this life. There are also levels moving downward from bad to worse, and finally to the worst. At any given point in time, each of us finds himself/herself somewhere within these ascending and descending stages leading into and out of the clinical netherworld. Like snowflakes, no one state of physical, mental, or spiritual existence is exactly like another; no two persons are ever at the same level. Dual medical procedures cannot be the mirror image of each other nor can the clinical outcomes. Some of these differences are morally relevant; some are not.

Life for all on the planet Earth virtually exists on the edge of a precipice, and the pathway to and from the edge is along an omnipresent slippery slope, requiring vigilance and perseverance to the very end. When confronted by the inner bravery of most who are significantly diseased, injured, or otherwise physically impaired, one has to ask: What is it within the human species that enables persons through the ages to overcome inestimable odds and to persevere in the face of life's most formidable challenges? Not only is this question related to humankind's struggle to live with and to overcome disease, injuries, and disabilities, it is applicable to all other serious tests that have been met and conquered by human beings in the course of their history. There is a biological and an apparent spiritual determinism in *Homo sapiens*, which is unique among the animals of the natural world.

Science, history, philosophy, and religion are replete with evidence of a flourishing spirit distinctive to humankind. This innate quality gives vitality to the most receptive parts of the mind, body, and soul and enables human beings to bear the unbearable and, innovatively, to reach out for the unreachable. Such spirit, often combined with faith and hope, is the pressing toward something that we anticipate achieving, or the overcoming of an obstacle or adversity that has confronted us. When faced with the problematic, it is this creative spirit that encourages human beings to be part of the solution. Philosopher/Theologian/Biologist Holmes Rolston, stated in his Gifford Lectures, *Genes, Genesis, God*:

> There appears, nascently in the higher animals and flourishing in *Homo sapiens,* a 'genius' or 'spirit' of extraordinary ingenuity and intelligence. In German, the term needed is *Geist.*[2]
> Environmental necessity is the mother of cultural invention . . . . All human culture, in which our classical humanity consists, originated in the face of oppositional nature. Nature insists that humans work, and this laboring and even suffering is its fundamental power for genesis. Creativity is through conflict and resolution. We suffer, and lest we suffer more, we organize ourselves creatively. . . . Suffering, far more than theory, principle, or faith, moves us to action. . . . Early and provident fear moves half the world. One should not posit the half-truth for the whole; we are drawn by affections as much as pushed by fears. These work in tandem reinforcement; one passes over into the other and is often its obverse. In this sense, pain is a prolife force. In the evolution of caring, the organism is quickened to its needs.[3]

Some years ago there was proliferating data documenting the number of individuals in the United States who had contracted HIV and who had subsequently developed AIDS. At that juncture twenty-five to thirty years ago, the disease bore with it a death sentence, longevity was not a realistic goal! As a deeply concerned pastor, I was a participant in the local AIDS-support group, Nashville Cares. An ecumenical worship service, at Christ Church Episcopal Cathedral in downtown Nashville, was held by the Cares organization to engender compassion and nurture for those who had been tragically infected with the disease. Persons of diverse religious and ethnic groups participated. It was well attended and was an unusually inspirational experience. At the conclusion of the service, a young man not more than twenty-one years of age, recognized me as one of several liturgists. Initially he acknowledged that, with no support group, he was a societal reject, without hope. Then he grasped my hand and, with tears forming in his eyes, said, "This was such an inspirational experience. Before this celebration I saw myself as a person *dying* with AIDS—but now I consider myself a person *living* with AIDS."

From that moment on, in my own professional and personal life, I recommitted myself to the compelling duty of lifting up those who demonstrate such remarkable courage in living with chronic/terminal disease, injury, or disability of any kind. Also, for similar reasons, most medical scientists have been tenacious in their research and have developed medications and procedures that are enabling that young man, and millions of others who rise above the netherworld shadows, to continue life with a reasonable hope for longevity and quality. The same level of commitment to find other cures and rehab enhancements for a multitude of medically compromised persons is occurring in research labs all over the world, and persons working in them remain inspired by individuals who display such courage.

Mary Helen Keller

We older Americans can benefit from a reintroduction to the life of Helen Keller. A new generation can benefit by getting to know about Helen Keller, perhaps for the first time. Though blind and deaf, she became one of the most famous persons in the entire world. Due to an unfortunate illness, she lost both her sight and her capacity for hearing at the age of nineteen months, giving a unique meaning to the descriptive "netherworld." Plunged into personal darkness by blindness and isolated from others by deafness, Helen's early emotional development gave way to animalistic forces within her unique shadowy existence. In her adult years she shared thoughts of the trauma that shaped her earliest memories:

> For nearly six years, I had no concepts whatsoever of nature or mind or death or God. I literally thought with my body. Without a single exception my memories of that time are tactual . . . there is not one spark of emotional or rational thought in these distinct, yet corporal memories. I was like an unconscious clod of earth. Then, suddenly, I knew not how or when, my brain felt the impact of another mind, and I awoke to language, to knowledge of love, to the usual concepts of nature, of good and evil.[4]

Deprived in early childhood of two of a human being's most important senses, hearing and sight, Helen's inability to grasp the significance of the most basic internal and external stimuli gave way to fits of rage and anger. Such behavioral response exhausted her family and herself. Then, when she was seven, the "miracle worker," Anne Sullivan, came into her life. Fortunately, her parents had the resources to enlist a special educator. Subsequently, this ingenious and devoted teacher and Helen developed a language with the combined senses of touch and the mind. It was the difference between abject darkness and unbounded light. Together with Anne, her constant companion from age seven and across many years, Helen learned English, German, French, Greek, and Latin through a Braille system, attended several preparatory schools for the blind, and entered Radcliff College at the age of twenty. After being graduated magna cum laude, she went on to claim the roles of author, lecturer, and activist in thirty-seven countries of the world. She lived thirty-two years past the death of her teacher and companion Anne Sullivan, during which time she displayed a remarkable capacity for independence within and beyond her limitations.

Mary Helen Keller was born in Tuscumbia, Alabama, on June 27, 1881 and died on June 1, 1968. In 1964 President Lyndon B. Johnson presented her with the Presidential Medal of Freedom, the highest civilian honor awarded to an American citizen. In 1999, *Time Magazine* issued a special edition honoring the 100 most important persons of the twentieth century. Helen Keller was one of them. In a commentary relative to Helen Keller and this award, famous jazz singer Diane Schurr (herself blinded in infancy) wrote, with Davis Jackson, "She altered our perception of the disabled and remapped the boundaries of sight and sense."[5] Later, in expressing her faith, Helen wrote,

> Once, affliction was looked upon as a punishment from God—a burden to be borne passively and piously. The only idea of helping the victims of misfortune was to shelter them and leave them to meditate and live as contentedly as possible in the valley of the shadow. But now we know that a sequestered life without aspiration enfeebles the spirit. It is exactly the same with the body. The muscles must be used, or they lose their strength. If we do not go out of our limited experience somehow and use our memory, understanding, and sympathy, they become inactive. It is by fighting the limitations, temptations, and failures of the world that we reach our highest possibilities.[6]

These are enlightened human desires that rise above and beyond mere instinctive capacities generic to all animal species, qualities abounding in *Homo sapiens* that suggest that the search for values such as beauty, truth, goodness, and achievement make this species unique above all others in the quest for a spiritual fulfillment—beyond the five physical senses—beyond mere biological survival—beyond the grim netherworld!

Mary Moore

All life begins and ends with struggle. "The 'birthing metaphor,' " writes Holmes Rolston, "is at the roots of the concept of 'nature'; here creativity comes only with 'labor' and 'travail.' "[7] At the outset, due not only to genetics but to environmental factors as well, many human beings experience physical adversity throughout their existence, and some succumb to early deaths. Although her quality of life at times would have been deemed to be poor, Chattanoogian Mary Moore persevered.[8] We have made reference to what might be called creative spirit, but with Mary, the characterization "indomitable" is applicable as well. Words, however, cannot explain the *Geist* of this winsome young woman. One had to meet her personally, see the bravery reflected in her eyes, notice her infectious smile, and listen to spirited words of faith and optimism for the future. When I walked into her room at Nashville's Vanderbilt University Medical Center one day in 1976, the first thing I noticed was a bumper sticker designed for automobiles but which she had attached to the metal foot of her bed: "Don't Bury Organs—Recycle Them!"

That Mary was very serious about this challenge to all was evidenced by the fact that she had been carrying the sign everywhere she went for three years following the complete failure of her kidneys in 1973 at the age of fifteen. Immediate dialysis was required three times a week at Erlanger Hospital in her home city of Chattanooga., Tennessee. There were numerous in-between visits to Vanderbilt, a distance of 240 miles round trip, until her successful transplant surgery there three years later.

After visiting Mary Moore at Vanderbilt, I could not erase from my mind the bumper sticker on the foot of her bed, "Don't Bury Organs—Recycle Them." Countless trips to Vanderbilt Medical Center from my church office in the Donelson community took me down Lebanon Pike to Fesslers Lane, into midtown Nashville and to Vandy. On the return trip after that first visit, the words on the sign still resonated. Suddenly there was a disturbing connection. As I turned onto Lebanon Pike from Fesslers, another sign, "Abernathy's Auto Parts," which I had passed innumerable times, took on an incongruous, yet relevant, aspect. Abernathy's is essentially an automobile graveyard. It is filled with wrecked cars. The link to Mary Moore unfolded as I continued slowly. Across Lebanon Pike and several hundred yards up the road from Abernathy's are two well-known Nashville cemeteries, Calvary and Mt. Olivet. The irony was the relationship of these cemeteries, not only to Mary's sign concerning human body parts, but also in their proximity to Abernathy's automobile graveyard. The automobile bodies were stripped of most of their usable parts while the human bodies were buried, the vast majority of them with significantly usable parts remaining.

The words "Don't Bury Organs" literally burned into my mind, my heart, and my conscience. Not long after that, my wife Judy and I effected a contract with Vanderbilt Medical Center to have our bodies, with all usable parts donated beforehand, sent immediately for medical research upon our respective deaths. Recently, due to our advancing ages, we concluded that our body parts would have less value for transplantation; so the entire corpses, will be sent to Vanderbilt University School of Medicine for cadaver lab use. In due time, a memorial service will follow for each of us. In a year or two, after that research is concluded, our bodies will be cremated and the cremains will be placed in the columbarium at Donelson Presbyterian Church, our present home for worship. Others, whom we know, are having all their usable parts stripped and donated at death through appropriate organ donation centers. Then, their bodies or cremains will be interred at cemeteries, columbaria, or other places of their choice.

In January of 1959, Mary Moore was born with a dislocated hip and a turned-inward right foot. Her hip was aligned by the age of six months. For two years she wore a metal brace connected between her two shoes to position her foot. Later, straps were attached to the right shoe and into a harness to help straighten her foot as she walked. These problems were essentially corrected between the ages of three and four. While in elementary school she was diagnosed with a progressive neurological malady, Charcot-Marie-Tooth Disease. Triple arthrodesis surgery was performed six months apart on each foot which corrected some of this condition:

> Charcot-Marie-Tooth Disease (CMT) is one of the most common inherited neurological disorders, affecting approximately 1 in 2,500 people in the United States. The Disease is named for the three physicians who first identified it in 1886. CMT, also known as hereditary motor and sensory neuropathy (HMSN) or peroneal muscular atrophy, comprises a group of disorders that affect peripheral nerves. The peripheral nerves lie outside the brain and spinal cord and supply the muscles and sensory organs in the limbs. Disorders that affect the peripheral nerves are called peripheral neuropathies.[9]

In 1969, when Mary was ten years old and still in elementary school, she was diagnosed with a kidney anomaly, glomerulonephritis. In spite of the latest available medicines and good medical care in Chattanooga and in Nashville at Vanderbilt, the disease grew worse. On a fateful day in 1973, total kidney failure occurred and dialysis was begun. This is the process of removing the urea and uric acid from the circulating blood, a necessary function usually accomplished by a normal kidney. Her mother remembers that, on the night before, Mary had gone with friends to eat pizza. It would be quite some time before she would eat pizza again, since her illness necessitated a controlled diet. Highly seasoned and exotic foods were a no-no! For almost three years she remained on the dialysis machines at Erlanger Hospital, dropped out of her ninth-grade public school and, when she felt up to it, received homebound tutoring.

The routine was an arduous one. Three days a week, six hours each of those days were required for the dialysis, along with an extensive daily regimen of assorted medications, in excess of twenty pills or capsules a day. Mary's mother, Peggy White, explained that persons on dialysis have varying degrees of toleration of the process. Some individuals get sicker than others from the dialysis routine. Mary was one of those who had a low capacity for endurance and, therefore, had to receive her treatments at Erlanger hospital instead of one of the freestanding dialysis clinics. Not only was Mary undergoing the blood purifying process on a regular basis, she was also receiving physical therapy at the Siskin Center in Chattanooga. This was a necessary response to the neurological and muscular problems with which Mary had struggled since early childhood, yet she persevered.

Other maladies plagued Mary, as well, during the three-year dialysis experience. At some point she developed what appeared to be appendicitis, thus requiring surgery during this vulnerable stage, periodically needing blood. Transfusions were considered 99 per cent safe. Ironically, Mary contracted malaria. Later, she struggled with pericarditis, an inflammation of the membranous sac surrounding the heart Then, as soon as she was sufficiently recovered from these setbacks, Mary was told that she could prepare for a trip to Nashville where she underwent thoracic duct drainage at Vanderbilt Medical Center. This procedure, accomplished under anesthesia, removed the lymphocytes from her body, which would have caused her to reject a new kidney if she were fortunate enough to receive one. In the 1970s it was a necessary pre-transplant requirement. In due time, as her condition improved, she was placed on the waiting list, a potential recipient for an organ transplant at Vanderbilt. There, on April 3, 1976, Mary Moore was implanted with an anonymously donated kidney flown in from somewhere in North Carolina. Her mother reported that alongside her smiling picture in the *Chattanooga News-Free Press,* was a caption with Mary's grateful response, "Someone else's generosity in death has given me a new start in life."[10]

At home again in Chattanooga, weeks passed and Mary's joy of being released from dialysis increased daily. Her extreme pleasure of being able to survive without the kidney machine was short-lived. Two months after the successful transplant at Vanderbilt, she was forced to return. Her ureter ruptured. The natural duct connecting the newly transplanted kidney to the bladder failed. Once more the urologists and nephrologists collaborated diligently to rebuild impaired body parts and save the new kidney. After a number of weeks, Mary was able to go home again and enjoy relatively good health.

During the late 1970s and early 1980s, Mary passed the General Educational Development exams, enabling her to receive her high school diploma and to enroll at Chattanooga State Community College. Subsequently she contracted influenza and was not sufficiently recovered for more than five weeks. Later, she transferred to the University of Tennessee at Chattanooga from which she was graduated. Prior to her graduation from the university, Mary had established a measure of independence by attending a driving school and learning to operate an automobile with the aid of manual controls. This was necessitated by the neurological disease that had forced her to rely on crutches in order to walk around the campuses as she attended classes.

In addition to completing college, Mary was able to travel within the USA, including Hawaii. It took special effort, but she traveled with her mother and her aunt to Israel and Egypt and, with her paternal grandmother, to Europe. She experienced a part-time employment opportunity with AAA (the automobile association) and volunteered for Christian outreach service through her church, Rivermont Presbyterian in Chattanooga. This congregation, and its pastor, Dr. Robert Watkin, Jr., rallied around Mary through all of the years of personal struggle. For them Mary was a symbol of courage and faith that they shared with others in the larger community. Her life story became a teaching tool for getting the organ transplantation challenge out to many in Chattanooga and elsewhere. At the same time, the extended church family was a source of inspiration and support, not only to Mary but to her courageous mother, Peggy White, and Peggy's supportive husband, Bill White. Both were absolutely committed to their daughter's best interest and well-being. One had to meet Peggy White, however, before fully understanding from whom Mary received her true grit, optimism, and personal faith.

In 1985 Mary Moore's kidney function began to decrease, a repeat of glomerulonephritis. Fortunately, she did not have to initiate dialysis that time; she was able to receive another successful kidney transplant in November of 1985, once again at Vanderbilt University Medical Center. She felt well until January 1986 when it was discovered that she had a growth in her sinus area. She returned to Vanderbilt Hospital where she underwent surgery to remove the tumor, which was feared to be malignant. It was, however, benign. Mary lost a significant amount of blood during the surgery, and preparations were made for additional transfusions. In the meantime, as she was being transported from surgery to recovery, she sustained a massive stroke. Never regaining consciousness, Mary died on January 15, 1986, two days following her twenty-seventh birthday. Retrospectively her mother, Peggy White, wrote:

> Mary had a strong Christian faith which really grew stronger with each medical problem that she lived through. Her family and friends in Chattanooga, and her minister, Dr. Robert Watkin, and the Rivermont Presbyterian Congregation were a tremendous support to her twenty-seven, all too short, years. It must be noted that if Mary had not had the excellent medical care available during those years, and the fact that God did answer many prayers for her, she would have lived a much shorter life. Thankfully, medical knowledge continues to improve each year, and more people are being educated to the need and importance of donating organs to give life to more individuals who otherwise would perish.[11]

Recently, I was visiting in the home of a beloved friend, Leon, who was dying with end-stage cancer and who was receiving home hospice care. To the end he was continuously surrounded by family and friends. Throughout, he was courageous and non-complaining. During one of my visits, I glanced toward the wall and hanging there was a piece of framed art work, cross stitched lovingly by one of his adult daughters. It was applicable to the Leons of the world, and to the Mary Moores. Interlaced with colorful birds, flowers, butterflies, and bumblebees was a brief caption, an interesting twist on the well-worn words in packaging, "handle with care." In this case the paraphrase stated, "Life is fragile–handle it with prayer." It is a universally documented fact that the physical vicissitudes of life drive most persons and their caregivers inward, through reflection or prayer, to tap the spiritual resources that are, according to Fosdick, "a natural function of human life . . . thus universal."[12]

Creative spirit seeks to unite with creative spirit when the five senses are intact—especially so when they are not, as evidenced in the life of Helen Keller. When one or more of the physical senses of sight, hearing, touch, taste, and smell are lost or adversely compromised in the human being, there generally is an effort on the part of the individual so impaired to draw on resources less emphasized, from dimensions within or beyond these five. This phenomenon is worldwide; it cuts across all religious boundaries and emerges in some form within every known culture.

Sections of the Catechism of Hinduism (in this case, Yajur Veda) refer to a liberating sphere beyond the physical, which is sought in *meditation*: "When cease the five (senses) knowledges, and the intellect stirs not, that, they say, is the highest course."[13] Buddhism, a highly syncretic religion, is replete within inner reflection. One source suggests that Buddhist meditation is fundamentally concerned with two themes: transforming the mind and using it to explore itself and other phenomena."[14] Islamic faith, springing from the Quran moves the individual beyond the temporal with its emphasis on the "five pillars" of the faith. One of the pillars is "Salat," a requirement that the adult believer face the east, kneel, and pray at five intervals through the course of a day.[15]

In ancient Hebrew literature, the prophet Isaiah proclaims, "but those who wait for the Lord shall renew their strength, / they shall mount up with wings like eagles, / they shall run and not be weary, / they shall walk and not faint"[16] In the Christian New Testament, the person and work of Jesus of Nazareth is a testimony to prayer and he taught his disciples not only the importance of prayer but, in turn, how to pray.[17] Paul of Tarsus, the apostle of Jesus, referred to the inner strength that comes from God, "We are afflicted in every way, but not crushed; perplexed, but not driven to despair; persecuted, but not forsaken; struck down, but not destroyed."[18] Later he encourages the church community gathered in first-century Thessalonica to "pray without ceasing!"[19]

Lorene Sharp White

Lorene Sharp was born on November 18, 1943, in Nashville at the Vanderbilt University Medical Center, the fourth child of Vernon Sharp, Jr., and Sarah Robinson Sharp.[20] Several years before Lorene's birth in 1943, the Sharp family moved from Nashville to 320 acres nearby in the picturesque Harpeth Valley of Williamson County in Middle Tennessee. Their new residence was an antebellum home named Harpeth, which had been built eighty years earlier in 1858 by a wealthy planter. Shortly before they were to move in, however, a tragic fire destroyed the main living quarters of Harpeth. Only the brick walls were left standing along with numerous outlying buildings.

Fortunately, the historic home was covered by insurance. Using the remaining brick walls of the charred former living quarters, the Sharp family built a stately mansion with seven bedrooms and named it Inglehame (home by the fireside), in tribute to their Irish ancestors. With a son, Vernon III, and two daughters, Sarah and Gertrude, already blessing their family, Vernon, Jr., and Sarah Sharp awaited the birth of their fourth child who would join the others in this picturesque setting. Among other things, there were red coats in the closets, stables for the horses, and kennel houses for the fox hounds.

But, beyond all other considerations for one of the most esteemed of Nashville area families, was the anticipated birth of another member of the family. She was the first child born within the family after their move to Inglehame, into a lifestyle that afforded every opportunity for a happy life, free of encumbrance.

Sarah Robinson Sharpe experienced a normal delivery in giving birth to her third daughter, Lorene, whom the family affectionately called "Renie." Weighing slightly more than seven pounds at birth, the baby and her mother remained in Vanderbilt Hospital for about ten days, an average stay following a birth in 1943. At the outset everything appeared to be normal. Gathered from family recollections and entries in her baby book, an early description of Renie stated, "She was a pretty baby, and showed an alertness and a level of activity that promised intelligence and character." But she just wouldn't eat. Later reports went on to explain that she did *eat*, "but only tiny incremental amounts." Within weeks, it was dreadfully apparent that Renie had serious problems.

Without the medical equipment available today, the family pediatrician, who had served the family well through the development of three other Sharp children, was at a loss to diagnose the problem. The other siblings had thrived in their infancy and early years of growth. In Renie's case, varieties of infant formulas were tried. As weeks passed, nothing seemed to be working. A family biographical account stated later, "Everyone knew that something was wrong, but no one knew what it was. The doctor admitted that he didn't have a clue." So, after several months, the physician declared that Renie was experiencing a significant, yet undiagnosed problem. Internal diagnostic capacities, catheterization, magnetic resonant imaging, and cardiac surgical procedures were not yet perfected. The family pediatrician had conscientiously done everything that his professional training and practice had taught him. He concluded that it was time to refer the case to someone else.

Rather quickly the Sharps located another physician who dedicated herself to the task of finding a reason for Renie's failure to respond to feeding efforts. A steady regimen of nutrition was vitally necessary for her sustained growth past infancy into childhood. However, it did not appear to be a digestive problem. Thus, struggling through the first eighteen months there was little change in the obvious fact that there was a disorder, the cause of which was yet to be determined. She was mentally alert, learning to walk and talk, and normally responsive at most other levels. There was some growth and weight gain, but she simply did not have the energy and stamina of a physically normal child. No one was offering a prognosis of longevity for Renie. One physician actually stated that she was "hopelessly ill."

In a May 1945 medical journal, Renie's physician read about a rare pediatric surgical procedure by Dr. Alfred Blalock that had taken place in November 1944 at Johns Hopkins Medical Center to correct a specific congenital heart defect. Subsequent procedures brought hope to many parents whose children had been born with a diagnosis of *patent ductus*, which is defined in part by the staff at Mayo Clinic:

> Patent ductus arteriosus (PDA) is a persistent opening between the major blood vessels leading from the heart. This heart defect present at birth (congenital) often closes on its own or is readily treatable. Left untreated, a patent ductus arteriosis can cause too much blood to flow through the heart, weakening the heart muscle and causing heart failure and other complications.[21]

One of the cardiologists collaborating with the pediatric surgeons at Johns Hopkins on the new heart procedures for infants, Dr. Helen Taussig, came to Nashville's Vanderbilt Medical Center to consult on an emergency case in January of 1946. In fact, the new *patent ductus* surgery was initially called the Blalock-Taussig procedure. Renie's pediatrician arranged for an examination of her young patient while the specialist was in the city. The Sharp family was elated. Dr. Taussig was the nation's leading diagnostician of heart problems in children. After a thorough examination, it was determined that Renie did, in fact, have symptoms of patent ductus arteriosus.

After a formal request to Dr. Blalock that she be accepted as a surgical patient, the date of May 7, 1946, was set for 2½-year-old Lorene Sharp's arrival by train in Baltimore at Johns Hopkins, under the care of her father and mother, Vernon and Sarah Sharp. Over several days there were numerous examinations, tests, needle sticks, and preparations, some quite painful and discomforting for a little girl who, much of the time, was separated from her parents. It was stressful, also, for the loving but anxious parents who, along with the physicians, would not know until completion of the surgery that the symptoms were confirmed. Immediately thereafter, the diagnosis came. She was indeed, in her early years, suffering from patent ductus arteriosus. The operation to alleviate that malady was a success. The news was spread with elation to the family and friends back home in Middle Tennessee.

For Vernon and Sarah Sharp, and later for other family and friends, the celebrations were abruptly short lived, however. The patent ductus situation had been corrected by the surgery and part of her physical distress was alleviated. Dr. Blalock assured them that there would be some better days ahead after Renie was sufficiently recovered from her surgery and hospitalization. But, he also told them that she would "never be a perfect baby." Stethoscopic examination after the surgery revealed that there was still a heart murmur that indicated an additional congenital problem. At that point in 1946 they had no way, short of surgery, of peering inside her body to be certain. With imaging technology and open-heart surgical possibilities still not perfected, once again, Renie's long term medical prognosis remained grim.

For a while she was able to do almost everything that her older siblings did. Yet, she was physically smaller than the others at the respective stages of their growth and could not match their energy levels. Even sister Margaret, the fifth child, who was born several years after Renie's hospitalization, soon outgrew her older sister in physical stature. At the same time, one could see in Renie an emergence of inner resources, genetically driven and, in her case, spiritually induced.

As a result, the years stretched beyond those prognosticated for Renie's early demise and in her adolescence she learned to ride a pony, subsequently larger animals, and on horseback had jumped the tallest fence on the estate. In due time, she was an enthusiastic participant in the foxhunts, which had become seasonal activities at Inglehame from the very first days of the family's move there. As Renie entered high school, however, her physical capacity began to wane significantly. Activities were selectively chosen. Fainting spells became commonplace, and she and her family were fearful and guarded, as were her classmates at school. During this stage of her life, Renie's need to pursue matters of faith and spiritual reflection also became important to her. Significant time, reflecting on her own mortality, was spent with her parish priest, the assistant cleric of the

Episcopal parish of which the family was a part. Renie desperately wanted to live and to contribute.

At some point near the time of her graduation from high school, Renie and her family were told by their new cardiologist at Vanderbilt that she had been born not only with patent ductus arteriosus but also with a hole in her heart, a malady called "Eisenmenger's Syndrome."[22] She underwent a new catheterization procedure, which confirmed that there was indeed a hole in the septum of her heart causing blood to leak between the two heart chambers that pumped blood to the lungs and to the rest of the body. The resultant pressure on the blood vessels of the lungs caused the blood vessels to thicken, and that resulted in a restriction on the flow of blood to the lungs and a concurrent reduction of oxygen to those vital organs, a crisis of significant proportion. The degenerative lung disorder was officially called pulmonary hypertension. If a repair of the septum defect were to be accomplished, a procedure that had become perfected by that time, a robust heart, pumping increased blood flow, would be an ominous threat to the compromised lungs that could no longer handle the volume. She was not expected to live past her teen years.

Her parents had been given such prognosis several times through the earlier years, but if Renie was aware of these dire predictions, this did not dissuade her from reaching out with "Geist" to overcome the limitations which she faced in growing up. Of such firmness of purpose, William Orton of Yale once wrote: "The will to live, the capacity to enjoy living, the strength to live well, are not the results of dialectic: they spring from the deepest biological roots, and rise with the active exercise of native impulse."[23]

Upon graduation from high school, Renie, ordinarily, would have gone to college at Sweetbriar in Virginia for two years and then back to Vanderbilt for the final two years and graduation. This had been the path of her older sisters, Sarah and Gertrude. But because of her physical limitations, Renie remained in Middle Tennessee and tenaciously spent six years studying at a slower but complete pace at Vanderbilt, and she experienced a relatively normal social life before graduating with a degree in history and art. After Vanderbilt, Renie embarked on a career in interior design, enrolling in courses with the New York School of Interior Design. She accomplished this through home study, followed by several weeks on campus in New York.

Completing the requirements of this program, Renie became associated with one of the leading Nashville companies of interior design.

Through these early years, however, Renie struggled with a desire to be involved in a career that would give her the sense of serving individuals through counseling, teaching, or some other spiritually fulfilling endeavor. Vocational guidance tests confirmed what she was inwardly feeling. She simply wanted to help other people. Her reflection led Renie to enroll at the Vanderbilt Divinity School, which she believed might ultimately give her a sense of direction and open the door to a fulfillment of her mission in life, service to others. She was twenty-seven years old.

It was at this point that civil engineer Raymond White and Renie Sharp became acquainted. They met at the swimming pool of the fashionable West End Nashville apartment complex in which they both lived, and they soon fell in love. Lorene Sharp, an Episcopalian, and Raymond White, a Presbyterian, were married. Raymond became a mainstay of comfort and support for Renie as she maneuvered through the demands and requirements of graduating from divinity school and preparing for ordination in the pastoral ministry, some facet of which would give her the opportunity to reach out in both a spiritual and social service.

The question remained as to which denomination would be the one of singular choice for the newly married couple. This was resolved by the fact that Presbyterians had already approved the ordination of women to the clergy. Episcopalians remained at the discussion level on that issue, permitting that ecclesiastical procedure a few years later. One of the requirements for ordination in the Presbyterian church was the study of Hebrew and Greek, the original languages of the Old and New Testaments respectively. Because of her physical constraints, Renie could have avoided this arduous study requirement, among others, by requesting ordination under the "extraordinary clause" in the Presbyterian Book of Church Order. This would have allowed her to follow a less physically strenuous and intellectually demanding pathway to her goal of ordination and service in the church. But Renie would not have it that way. Having already overcome so much in her young life, she cut herself no slack when it came to fulfilling the normal requirements, even if it took her a little longer to do it. The divinity school requirements ordinarily were accomplished in three years—for Renie it took four. She was one of the first two women ever to come under the care of the candidates' committee and the first to be ordained by Middle Tennessee Presbytery.

After her ordination, Renie continued her post-graduate training in counseling with a year's internship as a chaplain at Baptist Hospital in Nashville. She was also receiving some ominous signals about her health. Near Christmastime she began to experience heart arrhythmia, a further reminder to her of her fragile existence and her need be careful of the demands and responsibilities that were being laid upon her by her marriage, studies, examination, ordination, and the search for a place to serve in her new career.

Shortly after Renie completed the clinical pastoral program at Baptist Hospital, Donelson Presbyterian Church and this author entered the life of Lorene and Raymond White. On September 18, 1977, Renie White officially became a member of the staff of Donelson Presbyterian Church, and her husband, Raymond, became an active participant in the worship and work of the congregation. As Parish Associate, Renie first had responsibilities related to Christian Education, but she felt a compelling call to serve God directly through counseling individuals and couples. From that point on, Renie remained on the staff of Donelson Presbyterian, donating her time as an effective and beloved counselor, serving a constituency of both male and female singles and a number of married couples. Raymond White observed later:

> Very few persons ever realized the intensity with which she pursued her chosen ministry. She left behind her a trail of love, concern, and devotion that her peers have not forgotten. But even they didn't fully realize how much true grit the traveling of that trail required of her. She was driven by a desire to help others. Even though her life had been hemmed in by adversity, she was always conscious of the advantages she had and she was almost consumed by the need to repay. The fact that she was beginning to repay was lifting a great burden.

Shortly after Christmas 1980, as one burden was lifting, another one was falling upon Renie and Raymond White. Several episodes required that Renie become more dependent on oxygen for breathing, and one crisis placed her in the cardiac care unit at Vanderbilt. Her physician had indicated that the end was near, perhaps within months and no longer than two years. Further damage had been done, and her heart was slowly but surely collapsing. After the hospital stay, she was confined to home most of the time but still got around some in her wheel- chair accompanied by the portable oxygen tube upon which she had become dependent. Not one ever to give in to her limitations, Renie still received some counselees in her home after she was confined there

On September 5, 1981, Renie participated with a Roman Catholic priest in the wedding ceremony of a friend of Raymond's, who remembers it as her last official act as a Christian minister. Her condition was growing worse. After that, she seldom left the house and, a little later, rarely left her bed. On October 9, 1981, because of edema in her feet and ankles, and increasing difficulty in breathing, Raymond decided that it was time for Renie to return to the hospital, despite her protests. The situation was growing more grim each day. Then, suddenly, a ray of hope appeared. Dr. Norman Shumway, famous heart surgeon of Stanford University had returned to his alma mater, Vanderbilt University Medical School. In a symposium he lectured about Stanford's latest miracle operation, the heart-lung transplant. A new heart alone would have been no value to Renie. It would have overloaded her diseased lungs, and she would have died almost immediately. But the possibility of both a new heart and new lungs was a miracle waiting to happen.

Three months later, after a 112-day stay in Vanderbilt Hospital, in January of 1982 Renie and Raymond White flew to California and, upon landing, traveled to Stanford University Hospital. Renie anticipated prayerfully that she would soon be the recipient of a heart-lung transplant. Thousands of others, in behalf of Lorene, were praying for that as well. One person who arrived after Renie at Stanford for a heart-lung transplant was there only two days before acquiring a heart-lung transplant. The young man was the recipient of a transplant of both organs because organs became available that matched his physical requirements while Renie was waiting for hers. He did well afterward because the appropriate organs became available so quickly. After a year Renie was still waiting.

The primary reason for Renie White's long wait was the lack of national awareness of and response to the need for organ donations. Part of her problem, also, was that large lungs cannot be placed in small frames such as hers. The many variables—size, blood type, and other factors—must be coordinated for successful transplants. Coupled with the limited number of donor organs, the length of time waiting for any transplant is therefore completely unpredictable, even more so for one awaiting both heart and lungs. No one dreamed that the wait at Stanford would stretch out over such a long period of time. Again, the delay was not caused by Stanford Medical Center but rather by the inability of the donor system to produce organs that were compatible with Renie White's unique systemic requirements.

Waiting for a heart-lung transplant in California stretched out past the first year and into the next for Renie, still hooked to an oxygen generator and bedridden much of the time. After the first year of waiting, however, Renie wanted to go home for a visit. She had come to love many of her Stanford area friends, but she missed her family and friends back home. Her Stanford physicians saw no reasons why she could not make the trips. Raymond also had negotiated with American Airlines to keep an oxygen generator in Nashville, ready if Renie had to make an emergency trip to California to claim those precious organs if they became available. Actually, three visits to Tennessee were accomplished over the transplant waiting period as the time stretched out past twenty-two months.

The third trip back to Nashville was filled with excitement and nostalgia. They were going to spend Christmas 1983 at home. In the year before, the holidays in Menlo Park had been meaningful enough with their friends at the Valley Church and its pastor, The Reverend Lloyd Auchard. "It was as if," wrote Raymond later, "the star was not leading to Bethlehem but to Nashville, and we were going to follow it. The idea of actually being at home for that most wonderful of holidays glowed like a beacon."

On December 11, Renie and Raymond arrived in Nashville for a three-week visit. On Christmas Eve, with the temperature hovering near zero, colder than usual for Nashville, they went to the Donelson Presbyterian Church for the candlelight communion service. Though temporarily inactive, Renie remained on the staff and was still officially the Parish Associate. In his personal memoirs, Raymond later wrote:

> The church was decorated for Christmas with evergreen wreaths and swags around the walls, candles and poinsettia, and a Christmas tree covered with Christian symbols. The pews were rapidly filling with friends who were Christmas happy and who had not seen Renie for over two years. It was a good time to return. When Renie came in, dressed in her huge floor length red coat with me close behind lugging the oxygen tank, there was a flutter of excited pleasure throughout the congregation. Unexpectedly, here she was. After the service, people crowded around happily, and Renie was the center of a throng of devoted well wishers. Without enough breath to do much talking, she spent most of the time nodding and smiling. After two years of exile, during which she often worried that she had been forgotten, it was wonderful for me to see in their faces and hear in their greetings the truth that she had not been forgotten, and that she was loved now at least as much, if not more, than she had been before.

The next day, Christmas at Inglehame was like a page from one of Washington Irving's picturesque accounts of eighteenth-century Christmases in rural America. The setting was nearly perfect, and the entire Sharp family was gathered together for their Christmas meal and the sharing of gifts, the most precious of all being the presence of Renie and Raymond. From there it was a visit to the home of Raymond's Aunt Katherine where his family was gathered. Renie and Raymond left after a brief visit of half an hour; everyone knew that both were exhausted.

Remaining in bed on December 26, Renie was lovingly served a light mid-morning breakfast by Raymond, who then settled down in the nearby library with a book. A bit later he heard Renie's soft voice calling him, as she had so many times through the years, "Love, will you come in here!" She was sitting on the bedside. "It's my heart," said Renie. Her pulse began dramatic swings of acceleration and deceleration with accompanying seizure. Her body temperature spun out of control as well, inordinately high at one point and extremely low at another. It was a chaotic, nightmarish, netherworld moment.

Emergency services were immediately called, as were Renie's physicians at Vanderbilt University Hospital where she was born in 1943 and to which she was transported on that morning, the day after Christmas 1983. The monitor in the emergency service ambulance indicated that her heart stopped beating three or four minutes before her arrival at the Vanderbilt trauma unit. Within a few minutes more she was resuscitated and a damaged brain coalesced with a dramatically failing heart. At 3:00 a.m. on the next morning, December 27, Renie was pronounced dead.

The legacy of The Reverend Lorene Sharp White, as that of Mary Moore, is a testimony to many in this life who contend with chronic disease and impairment. Though living at the edge on a daily basis, to the very end she never gave up. Renie existed in a state of hope—patiently waiting for a heart-lung transplant—never giving in to despair. Her tenacity and faith are a challenge to all, that we have a societal obligation to render support to those among us who start every day physically and mentally challenged. It is also a reminder to us that within every human being there is a potential resource and strength which, at least for a period, can offset many of life's adversities.

Chapter III

Overcoming the Netherworld

Claiming a Good Death

In due time, the sparrow falls to the ground. Sooner or later the natural world claims its own. With the human species, death is often perceived as an accident or illness, and as such potentially becomes an enemy. But death is not always the enemy. At times it may arrive as a friend, at a time when the human body no longer serves its purpose as the earthly dwelling place of the soul. When the biological systems of the body fail, death arrives and with it comes the cessation of pain and oft-times the unending and overwhelming physical and mental discomfort. In that sense, death may be perceived as a good. The last gasp of air and its subsequent release from the body is somewhat like a final great sigh of relief as the physical mass gives itself up. The potentially harrowing netherworld experience is brought to its natural conclusion. A significant value of seeing a loved one laid out in a funeral home casket, or even on a funeral pyre, is the comforting sense of peace that encompasses the corpse. A similar value may embrace those interring the ashes of a loved one in an urn or spreading them in a location of special meaning to the deceased and/or the family and friends.

Contrasting scenarios are those when a body cannot be found, as being lost at sea, when blown apart by an airplane explosion at thirty-six thousand feet above the earth, when devastated by a Caribbean earthquake, or when swept away by an Asian tsunami. Sudden natural disasters frequently strike with such magnitude that respectful individual burial procedures necessarily give way to mass interments accomplished with the aid of bulldozers and front-end loaders. The course of dying itself, therefore, is not always predictable nor is it necessarily manageable or peaceful. When we talk about desiring a good death, we are ordinarily talking about mitigating the process of dying rather than focusing on death itself. Oftentimes, the prelude to death is surrounded by carnage and ugliness as in war, natural disasters, or wanton societal greed and neglect. It is such horror and turmoil that we are hoping to prevent at the end of life, but which many times are inescapable. Even in the sanctity of home or hospital, the final moments of life before death arrives may be accompanied by rather bizarre manifestations of physical, mental, and emotional trauma.

The setting in the bedroom of Renie and Raymond White was confused and disordered when her heart functions spun out of control. The situation at the hospital was not any more serene when the physicians attempted by resuscitation to wrest control of Renie's life from the hands of death. In Raymond's account of his beloved's final hours, he writes descriptively:

> When she was settled in her room, I went to see her and then, in ones and twos, everyone else went in to see her to say goodbye. It was not a pleasant scene. The respirator tube was down her throat, taped in place and every few seconds the machine gave her chest a violent heave. The inevitable IV fluids were dripping and she was attached to the heart monitor. All those lifesavers that had worked before weren't going to pull it off this time. She was unconscious, yet her disordered brain had her eyes open, darting looks wildly about the room, and her hands were randomly twitching. It was appalling. The Renie we knew was already dead and the thought that went through almost all of our minds was a prayer that she wouldn't have to go through this very long.

Such a dramatic and soulful episode forces us to reach out once more to examine the meaning of the Greek noun *euthanasia*. My lexicon tells me that this word is a combination of two others. The word "eu" (meaning good, well, easy, friendly, or kindly disposed) is prefixed to the word "thanatos" (meaning death). The word *euthanasia* has been used actively as in mercy killing and passively as in allowing to die. Most of us would hope for a "good death," one that comes in a friendly or "kindly disposed manner," a process that is brief and easy, one that is without labor or effort. Realizing, however, that this type of death does not always occur, we should not be dissuaded from seeking such when the possibilities exist for it.

That is the purpose of advance directives and of hospice care with its emphasis upon comfort and upon palliation. The French, in their practice of fifteenth-century medicine, coined a pithy folk expression that lies at the heart of today's hospice movement and is relevant to the current emphasis on comfort care in the contemporary hospital: "Guerir quelquefois, soulager souvent, consoler toujours," which, Anglicized, affirms, "to cure sometimes, to relieve often, to comfort always."[1]

In the course of events that unfold in the hospital, the hospice, the nursing home, or the private residence, there is invariably the prognosis that little or nothing more can be done medically to effect a cure or to stave off death in specific cases. Through the years, as pastor and clinical ethicist, I often heard professional caregivers grimly utter to family members the phrase that no one wanted to hear, but that was commonplace at the bedside, in the hall outside the patient's room, or at the nurses' station: "There is nothing more that we can do." Many in these clinical settings, however, affirm that there is often more that *can* be done—palliative care—the mitigation of pain and the alleviation of physical discomfort.

It is vital, therefore, that we see the subtle distinction between *treatment* and *care* in the clinical setting—to acknowledge the physician or nurse, not only as a technician but as a professional with values. John Peppin, D.O., has written an insightful article, which is helpful here in dealing with this difference. "Empathy, sympathy, compassion, and care are expressions of deeply held beliefs and values. Even the language used to define these terms is value laden."[2] At Summit Medical Center in Nashville, I served on the staff as Consultant in Medical Ethics and Director of the Center for Clinical Ethics. A memorandum was circulated through the hospital channels by the Institutional Ethics Committee of which I was chairman. We were in the process of writing a new "Futile Care Policy and Procedure," crafted on principles recommended by the American Medical Association Council on Ethical and Judicial Affairs.[3] Several days later, I was confronted in the hallway by the Director for Human Resources, Perry Stahlman. In a very kind but professional way he asserted, " 'Treatment' may be futile but attempts to 'care' never are!" When our ethics committee concluded its meeting, the name on the new policy and procedure was subsequently entitled: "The Futile Treatment Policy" rather than "Futile Care Policy."

While the efforts *to cure* may appear to be elusive, one might assume that the least thing caregivers can do in seeking the "good" of the patient, is to *relieve often* and *comfort always.* The colloquial response is, "that may be easier said than done." University of Texas Cancer Center Physician Stratton Hill has been among those in the medical profession who are clamoring for better results in pain management. A decade and a half ago he raised the question: "When will adequate pain treatment be the norm?" Then he argued, "Inadequate treatment of pain continues to be a problem." Commensurately he observed, "Medical school curricula are woefully lacking in teaching medical students treatment of acute pain and the complexities of chronic pain treatment."[4] That was in December of 1995.

One would assume, again, that such concerns have been addressed by now and that improvements in pain management education have been implemented, not only in medical and nursing schools but also through continuing education for professional staffs in hospitals and medical centers throughout the country. In May 2008 one pain management symposium at Yale School of Medicine, however, took a prompting from the Joint Commission on the Accreditation of Healthcare Organizations and reaffirmed: "In recent years, pain has been designated as one of the vital signs indicating a patient's well-being." The published report also stated, "Yet only 3% of the nation's medical schools, including Yale, currently have a separate course in pain management."[5] On April 29, 2011, an online editorial by the International Association for the Study of Pain suggests that pain management and education remain highly complex issues:

> Although most formal decisions as to the management of pain are made by doctors, it has been obvious for a long time that medical undergraduate teaching on the subject of pain leaves much to be desired. Many medical schools teach very little about pain at either the preclinical or clinical levels and information is poorly integrated. Changing medical undergraduate curricula is never an easy task. It is one which needs to be catalyzed and facilitated in a variety of ways.[6]

One major impediment in aggressively treating pain, while trying to treat a disability or cure a disease, is the use of opioids and other narcotics. Most health-care professionals have concern about the addictive nature of such drugs. Medical professionals, including ethicists, have termed the phenomenon of addiction as one which should be addressed always with deliberation, caution, and vigilance when prescribing and treating long-term medical anomalies and when impending death is not an issue.

End-of-life care is another matter. When imminent death is a factor, along with others I would argue that concern for addiction is a moot point—an overriding moral priority for the dying patient should be *relief* and *comfort*.[7] However, the regimen of opioids and other narcotics for such unquestionably moral purposes also bears with them the unintended consequence of respiratory depression. The use of such substances may accelerate by hours or days the moment of death, and have been termed "double effect." Eric Raefsky, M.D., oncologist at Nashville Summit Medical Center contends:

> The vast majority of cancer patients will experience pain during the course of their disease. Indeed, the World Health Organization has recognized uncontrolled pain as a significant problem in many cancer victims. For this reason, narcotics are being prescribed in a majority of patients. Several obstacles, including patient and physician reluctance to use drugs with abuse potential, have limited their optimal use. Most ethicists agree that these medicines should not be withheld from terminal patients due to fear of their addicting potential. However, concerns about possible side effects, notably hypotension and decreased respirations, often lead to discontinuation of these medicines when patients are actively dying. From an ethical viewpoint, this is difficult to justify. While most American ethicists do not believe in active euthanasia, they are willing to accept the possible side effects of medicines given for relief of symptoms. As the goal of narcotic use is to alleviate pain, anxiety and agitation that often accompanies the dying process, they should not be withdrawn when

needed most in fear that they may shorten life by hours or days. While that may be a possible side effect, that risk is easily justified when quality of life issues become paramount.[7]

Heroic treatment in the clinical setting may be deemed futile and may be withdrawn. But, the Human Resource Director at Summit was absolutely correct, comfort and care should not cease until death has been medically confirmed. As long as there is life in the patient, and resources are available, compassionate care should be expended to mitigate pain, to alleviate discomfort, to preserve dignity, and to be a reassuring presence. My former clinical colleague, Dr. Bruce White[8] insists that three things are the minimum for palliative care in the hospital to ensure: (1) that the patient is in a clean bed, (2) that the patient is as free from pain and discomfort as is medically possible, and (3) that the patient is placed in an environment where family, friends (and perhaps even pets) can be present as with many hospices, institutional and home. This community of support, large or small, is critically important in a society where the aging population is dramatically increasing and where they, and many singles of varying ages, live in isolation and loneliness.

As our nation's aging, debilitated, and dying populations increase, many are suggesting that we need to concentrate our efforts on psychosocial aspects of health care with vigor equal to that of the medical model. In a recent interview, physician Robert L. Martenson stated,

> Most Americans die in hospitals or nursing homes, and neither is configured to take care of dying patients. There's little palliative care available and often the payment structure of health insurance doesn't support it. So you end up with situations where a 90-year-old with organ failure is brought to the emergency room and the doctors go "Let's tune her up." Or if the patient starts failing at the nursing home, they'll say, "No one dies here. Let's get her to the emergency room." It is not unusual in the last six months of a patient's life that they'll be shuttled between the nursing home and the hospital 6, 8, 10

times and subjected to a lot of painful and expensive interventions. The patient is maintained that way until the body gives out.[9]

Increased plans must be made for hospitals and health-care delivery staff who are equipped with the hospice modality to counter this "revolving door syndrome"—to meet the needs of those seeking more hospitable settings within which persons of any age may spend their final days. Hospice type institutions and home care have existed in countries beyond our shores for many years. As a matter of fact, over the last several decades national concerns for palliative and comfort care have led to the addition of hospice units to acute and chronic care hospitals in most areas of this country. More will follow, with increasing emphasis simultaneously upon homebound hospice care.

Above all, we must concentrate on the individual's sense of personal worth and provide assurances to an aging community or to persons of any age, that individual lives have value and that they are cherished. Then and only then, will we as a society turn our aging population and our lonely singles away from the despairing notion that suicide or mercy killing are the exits of first or only resort when faced with debilitating illness and or incurable diseases near the end of life. In the interview with Dr. Martenson, Claudia Dreifus of *The New York Times* asked, "Can there be such a thing as a good death." The physician responded, "My father had one." He then proceeded to cite the withholding of technologies and procedures that would have extended life but that offered no cures. "My father died comfortable, surrounded by people who loved him."[10]

Ruth Stanley[11]

All end-of-life experiences do not result in oppressive life-support systems, litigation, or thoughts of self-delivery. As many have suggested, there are alternatives, ones which the family of Ruth Stanley astutely embraced. This diminutive eighty-seven-year-old lady had made known her wishes concerning her own exit from life. "I don't want a bunch of tubes. I've had a full life," she had told her daughter Joan several times. "I don't want to be kept alive if I can't be up and useful to somebody. I don't even want to be a burden to my children. To be in bed or to sit in a chair and have to be fed and waited on isn't living. Please, if you can do anything about it, don't let me stay around like that."

A native of Columbus, Ohio, Ruth, in her later years spent about half of her time visiting a daughter Ruthie in California and about half of her time with her daughter Joan who was a retired registered nurse in Nashville, Tennessee. Occasionally, she would also visit her son, Jack, who lives in Oregon. In 1987, after hearing that she had suffered a massive stroke in Nashville, I (Joan's pastor) arrived at the hospital bedside and found her paralyzed on her left side, barely conscious, and unable to eat, even with assistance. It appeared that her life was nearly over.

After a week or so she was transferred to a nursing care medical unit where her daughter Joan and I met initially with the head nurse and then the administrator. They could not find veins for feeding we were told, so she would have to be given liquid food and water through a feeding tube. Such policy and procedure were universal medical protocol for that institution. They had already placed her in a double room with a ninety-one-year-old woman who had been there for two years in fetal position and kept from dying by antibiotics and a feeding tube. The roommate's activity consisted of being bathed and turned to prevent bedsores and of being fed through the tube. That endless cycle was broken three times, however, when she was taken to the hospital with pneumonia. "After that," said Joan, "She would be brought back to the nursing home to vegetate some more."

Mrs. Stanley's daughter Joan had heard the staff describe the roommate's situation and knew that neither she nor her mother would want her to be subjected to a similar routine. "Mama doesn't know anybody," said Joan. Then she added, "She made little or no response to our promptings. So, we decided we'd bring Mama home." A succinct observation by Eric Cassells is appropriate here: "The right medical practice will provide those who may get well with the assistance they need and it will provide those who are dying with the care and assistance they need in their final passage. To fail to distinguish between these two sets of medical practice would be to fail to act in accord with the facts."[12]

The daughter Ruthie from California and son Jack from Oregon came to be with Joan and their mother during what they knew would be their parent's final days or weeks. Alive Hospice of Nashville, a non-profit agency dedicated to home and institutional care of terminally ill patients, was called to assist. They set up a hospital bed, sent in nurses periodically, and pledged to locate sitters if needed. They were two sisters and a brother to deliver loving care for their mother in her dying moments, so it was not necessary to hire the sitters. The prognosis was that Ruth Stanley was terminally ill; she had six months or less to live. Therefore, Medicare payments were transferred to Alive Hospice for the home care of the patient during the last stages of her life.

Separately, Joan shared the story with a medical reporter for the now defunct *Nashville Banner* and with me, her pastor, in hope that others might be given new insights concerning alternatives at the end-of-life. She desired also that others would take charge of their own destiny or that of loved ones seeking to fulfill requests similar to those that earlier Mrs. Stanley had requested of them. Ruth Lakin Stanley died two weeks after coming home, in the manner she had sought, with dignity and surrounded by love. Joan shared with me an account of the final days for other caregivers in similar situations to consider:

> The feeding tube had been removed at the medical unit of the nursing care center. We brought her home and placed her in bed. We gave her ice chips when she seemed up to it. We talked to her every time we turned her, touched her with love—-and she did respond, until whispering her adult children's names, she lapsed into a final coma. After she had greeted each of us—and knew she was home—she was ready to go.

These siblings made their decisions concerning the end of life of their mother based on the conversations which they previously shared with her and the physicians and nurses associated with Alive Hospice, along with full pastoral support. These poignant discussions, including their mother's own verbalized advance directives, enabled them to celebrate the relationships that they were privileged to enjoy in the time allotted their family. There were no denials or delusions concerning the finiteness of life. In many ways they were among the fortunate who have come to terms with the value of human life, the joy of relationships, and the fact that these gifts are held in earthen vessels. At the end, their decisions spared them the final moment of death occurring in the oppressive technological ethos and moral complexity of the clinical netherworld. For everyone lovingly concerned, it was a good death!

Chapter IV

Playing God

Some years ago, the chief of the medical staff in a Nashville hospital, a general surgeon, approached me in the physician dining room. This setting was conducive to private discussions among physicians and other staff regarding patients whom they were mutually attending. As the staff clinical ethics consultant, I was welcomed to this dining area by the medical and administrative staff, a non-physician along with a few others, including the hospital chaplains. A patient of this surgeon was dying of cancer and lay in an unresponsive comatose state in one of the hospital rooms upstairs. Two sons and a daughter-in-law gathered faithfully for several weeks at his bedside. Though physically devastated from the ravages of the malignancy that spread to his brain, the patient's cardio-respiratory functions were relatively stable and resistant to the final throes of death.

When the surgeon saw me enter the dining room, he motioned for me to go with him to a less busy area where we could have an uninterrupted conversation. Earlier that day this physician had visited the room of his patient. At that time, comment was made by the physician to the family gathered in the room that the end was near, but that the patient's heart function was surprisingly strong and was essentially staving off death. Unexpectedly, one of the sons lovingly raised the question of the heart pacemaker, which the physician had replaced some months earlier with a new one. "If the heart function is about all that is keeping our dad from dying, why can't you just remove the pacemaker or simply turn it off?" The question was a simple one, yet profound, as was the query of the physician a bit later in the dining room: "Can I morally and legally do that?"

Before I was able to make any kind of response, the physician informed me that the patient's cancer was inoperable and that one day in the not too distant future he would die from the disease. But he did cherish having several more months with his family, if able to sense their presence. At that earlier moment in the office, the patient mentioned to his physician that near the end he would not want aggressive or heroic measures attempted. The physician said also that he glanced briefly at the advance directive to that effect in his patient's chart in the office.

"Let me ask you several questions," I said to the surgeon. "Did you record in the chart your conversation with the patient earlier in the office?"

"As a matter of fact, I did," he responded.

"Well, then," I said," "do you accept the ethical and legal precept that a patient or his surrogate has the right to refuse treatment."

"Yes, definitely!"

"Do you believe that a patient or his surrogate has the right to request withholding or withdrawing a respirator or a feeding tube when there is no commensurate medical benefit?"

"Of course," he responded once more.

"Then, why not a pacemaker? It has value only in maintaining a relatively normal status quo. You of all people certainly know it has no capacity for cure. In this case it may be more of a burden than a benefit."

"I think I have my answer," he said with a smile.

"The bottom line," I added, "is that patient autonomy and the right to refuse treatment are relevant here. Not only do you have the patient's advance directive in your chart, you have the briefly recorded comments made in your office several months ago. Furthermore, when the patient no longer had decision-making capacity, his son, the legal surrogate, requested that his dad be allowed to die without the continuation of aggressive treatment, as indicated in his advance directive."

After lunch that day, a cardiologist came to the room of the dying patient and, in concert with the general surgeon, deactivated the pacemaker. Within several days the patient died peacefully. The underlying cause of death was advanced cancer. The pacemaker synchronized the heart rhythm but only prolonged the eventual outcome; the removal of the technology allowed imminent death to happen. Such decisions are rightly facilitated within the patient/physician relationship. Throughout, this patient and physician were of one mind regarding the eventual outcome. The compassionate physician maintained their fiduciary relationship, even though the patient had lost the capacity of awareness. The patient's trust in the covenant, made beforehand, was honored—morally delivered under the rubric "allowing to die."

Later that day the nurse supervisor on that floor paged me and asked me to meet with her concerning the removal of the pacemaker on that floor of the hospital. It seems that, afterwards, two of the nurses in that unit had engaged in a heated discussion at the nurses station as to whether or not this had been a case of the physician and the family "playing God!" My response to the nurse supervisor was that the physician was no more playing God when he shut down the pacemaker than he was at the outset of the initial placement of the tiny instrument just below the surface of the skin on the upper chest.

The nebulous but frequently used phrase "playing God" has been affixed through the ages to a variety of human endeavors. The label has been applied many times in history when scientists were on the verge of dramatic breakthroughs into biological, geological, and cosmological dimensions previously not broached. In this present age of in-vitro fertilization, recombinant DNA, cloning, stem-cell research, genetic engineering, gene therapy, screening and splicing, many are questioning what medical scientists should or should not be doing in their systematic inquiry.

How far, medically and legally, should they be allowed to go? When, where, and by whom should they be stopped? Who decides? Medical technologies are firmly established as treatments of choice at the clinical bedside. How do we respond to the charges that physicians, nurses, and other caregivers are routinely playing God in withholding of respirators or withdrawal of feeding tubes and other technology in the clinical netherworld?

As we have just seen, the expression "playing God" is thus part of the conversation that surfaces from time to time at the clinical bedside, in the hospital waiting rooms, and in homes across the nation. At the nursing stations and nearby consultation rooms, healthcare professionals gather to scan and discuss patient charts, pursuant to negotiation of treatment plans with patients and their families. Seldom, if ever, have I heard the term "playing God" used by professional or lay caregivers when physicians, nurses, and technicians *initiate* the treatment of diseased or seriously impaired human beings with the intent of seeking improvement or a cure. At the first mention of *withholding or withdrawing* treatment, however, the negative implications and use of the phrase "playing God" often surface. In my opinion this knee-jerk double standard is not morally valid for the clinical setting.

The use of technology, in and of itself is not the issue. The essential question is: When and under what set of circumstances should a medical procedure be initiated in the first place? For good or ill, a medical procedure is an interference with the natural process. Everything depends on the medical indications that initially warrant the procedure. I would argue that, if we are going to accept responsibility for *introducing* a beneficial medical procedure, then we must likewise accept or claim the responsibility for *withholding and withdrawing* non-beneficial medical support. If applicable to the withholding or withdrawal of a medical procedure, the phrase "playing God" itself is equally relevant to the process of initiating a medical procedure in the first place. As for me, if some persons want to use that terminology in either case, I will sanction that label responsibly, because I believe that is precisely what God wants me to do when medically appropriate.

If driven by the oft-used sanctity of life or medical vitalist principle of saving life at all costs, technology can become an unquestioned tool valued for its capacity to salvage bodily function, even when confronting overwhelming scientific evidence suggesting futility. "In our minds, at least, technology is always on the verge of liberating us from personal discipline and responsibility," wrote John Naisbitt three decades ago. Also, warning us against a "technofix mentality" he adds, "Only it never does and it never will."[1]

Recently, I saw a caption on an outdoor church sign that was intriguing and relevant to this discussion. As if to counteract the charge of playing God, it stated simply: "God's part we cannot do—our part God will not do." In our responsibility at the geological, biological, and cosmological levels of human existence, we must not evade our creative birthright by placing the complex issues of survival back into the hands of God to manage. Professor Maguire expresses a similar thought: "Made in the image of the Creator-God, we are by destiny creative. We may of course fail that destiny, but the Christian views himself (herself) as a co-creator, co-provider, and trusted steward within the kingdom. Christian genius and work must not be seduced into an adulterous union with the status quo."[2]

At some point in the 1950s while in theological seminary in Richmond, Virginia, I was introduced to the helpful book entitled *The*

Meaning Of Prayer, written by the great Baptist minister of the early twentieth century, Dr. Harry Emerson Fosdick.[3] It was that book, first published in 1915, which convinced me in later years that many of the complex decisions made by people of struggle and faith are not at all dynamics of playing God but rather dynamics of *cooperating* with God, as suggested by Dr. Maguire. In matters of beginning-of-life, end-of-life, and critical issues in between, God has placed in our hands the natural capacity to be creative. It is our biological and spiritual birthright!

In his book, Fosdick essentially makes the point that we cooperate with God in at least three ways—"by thinking, by working, and by praying"[4]—and that one of these can never be a substitute for the other. Then he suggests how wonderful it would be if we could simply swing our bridges into place with a prayer, which of course, we cannot. We must use our minds to design them, our hands to build them, and our prayers to acknowledge that it was God who gave us these creative abilities in the first place. One cannot abridge or ignore the laws of nature, but we can work within those laws, using them with dramatic and self-fulfilling consequences, even within the somber bowels of the clinical netherworld.

Unfortunately, moral innuendos of suicide and assisted suicide are tossed about at a variety of levels relative to such decisions along with the somewhat derogatory phrase of playing God. There are still nagging ethics questions in this country, among the physically disabled, the medical and religious enthusiasts, and many others, on withholding and withdrawing life-support systems. This holds true, even though Congress passed the Patient Self-Determination Act in 1990, to become effective in 1991.[5] The U.S. Supreme Court ruled in 1996 that a competent patient has a right to refuse medical treatment.[6]

Much earlier, mainstream religious groups had responded to the ethical and faith issues involved in allowing persons to experience a natural death. They deemed these actions to be cooperating with God, not playing God. The U.S. Catholic bishops, at their National Conference in 1994, reaffirmed an Ethical and Religious Directive for Catholic Health Services, which initially in 1981 stated: "A person may forgo extraordinary or disproportionate means of preserving life. Disproportionate means are those that in the patient's judgment do not offer a reasonable hope of benefit or entail an excessive burden, or impose excessive expense on the family or community."[7] However, the "extraordinary" clause cited by the bishops, did not include nutrition and hydration, considered rather to be "ordinary" measures, which they believe should be continued, as we shall see later in this manuscript.

A policy statement adopted by the merged 200th General Assembly (1988) Presbyterian Church (USA), said in part:

> When life support systems are removed, after reasonable and responsible attempts to save have run their course, allowing death to complete it course, we must not confuse that acknowledgement of death with the taking of life. We must be clear about the difference between killing and allowing to die. In our faith understanding, when the capacity for human relationship is irretrievably lost, death has occurred regardless of what biological function can be sustained.[8]

Commenting several years after life-support withdrawal and death of her own daughter, the mother of one ALS patient expressed to me the wish: "that all patients had the opportunity to make the decisions that she was able to choose for herself. I believe that the control my daughter felt helped her enter her dying experience with less fear—in her own time."

To be able to exercise such an opportunity to negotiate one's end-of-life process may not make the decision any easier, however. Perhaps one could assume that no one of sound mind and spirit capriciously makes the arbitrary decision of leaving this life for a destination from which no one returns. Emphatically, we should be of every encouragement and moral support for those who choose to continue life within enfeebled or disabled states. On the other hand it is grossly unjust to patients in horribly debilitated conditions to insist that they remain locked in to a terminally ill state with poor quality or no quality, against their wishes and the wishes of their families. The major difference is that many persons in these terribly diminished latter states are languishing at the point of death or have arrived at states in which their very personhood is disputable—it is not a matter of courageously *living* within one's limitations or disabilities.

Being able, legally, to choose the time of one's death and having the opportunity to do so are nevertheless two significantly different things. Sherwin B. Nuland, M.D., expands on that fact. This professor of surgery and of the history of medicine at Yale writes: "For too many of us, the manner of death will prove to be beyond control, and no knowledge or wisdom can change that."[9] Dr. Nuland realistically echoes scientists, poets, theologians, and others preceding him who have expressed a similar point of view on the fickleness and uncertainty of life and death. Patient autonomy may suggest at least some limited control, but some decisions about our own death may lie beyond our individual capacity to orchestrate.

The first-century Roman philosopher Seneca asserted, "Just as I choose a ship to sail in or a house to live in, so I choose a death for my passage from life."[10] Initially, Seneca and Dr. Nuland appear to be in agreement, i.e., persons leave this life in many different ways. But, Nuland qualifies his statement: "The great majority of people do not leave life in a way they would choose." In other words, the natural world oft-times does its own thing, in its own way, at its own time; more than likely it does not allow choice. When it does come and we may not be of sound mind, it might behoove us in advance to execute directives that give us a semblance of choice.

Subsequently, that places Dr. Nuland in discord with Seneca because the ancient philosopher supplements his statement by suggesting that leaving life is a matter of choice, the opposite of that which the Yale physician stated."[11] Obviously Seneca is referring to suicide as an arbitrary way out of this life, if the way be clear at some designated point. Suicide is precisely *not* what Dr. Nuland is discussing or advocating—*nor* is it the purpose of this book, which is to plan ahead for one's death and to plan it well, when natural circumstances permit such choice.

Many have followed with hope the aggressive use of new medicines, procedures, and technologies in health care—the seeking of ultimate solutions to the manifold problems of disability and disease throughout life at its beginning and end. Therefore, we should never cease to applaud the faceless men and women of science who labor through the centuries in laboratories worldwide to provide countless and sometimes dramatic breakthroughs leading to extended life and quality of life. Among countless others, some of the pioneers who persevered and achieved fame in specific areas of research, along with the gratitude of the people of the world are: Hippocrates, 460-377 BC (Greece).; Galen c130-200 AD (Asia Minor); Later stalwarts leading into the era of modern medicine: Englishman, Jenner, (small pox); Japanese, Kitasato (tetanus); Frenchwoman, Curie (radium therapy); German, Koch (tuberculosis, anthrax, surgical infection); Italian, Grassi (malaria); Austrian, Landsteiner (blood-type classification and transfusion); Frenchman, Pasteur (rabies, pasteurization, surgical infection); Frenchman, Laennec (stethoscope); Russian, Metchnikoff (typhoid fever); American, Reed (yellow fever); German, Rontgen (X-ray); American, Lauterbur, Englishman, Mansfield (Magnetic Resonance Imaging); Italian, Riva-Rocci (blood pressure cuff); Scotsman, Fleming and Australian, Florey, et al, (penicillin); American, Dickson, (band-aid); Americans, Kuhl and Edwards, (CT scan); American, Salk (polio); Englishmen, Hounsfield and Cormack (PET scan); American Drew, (plasma, blood bank); American Emerson and American Bird, et al., (ventilator); Frenchman, Montagnier and American, Gallo (AIDS). The research is ongoing and new breakthroughs lift our expectations for manifold cures and resurgent quality of life.

So, after having discovered so much about life and its processes, there is much more that we do not know. We are not infinite, though our basic inner struggle and natural capacity for survival at times lulls us into believing that perhaps we are! Scientific progress only exacerbates the delusion. Quality of life incrementally improves for some while, at the same time, progressively diminishes for others. Life's parameters are continually stretched, but countless humans still experience accidents and disease every second of every day. Emerging human beings, crawling around in dark prehistoric caves, faced their own sense of finitude when, in contrast to the lower animal species, they gradually became aware of the fact that one day they would die. The remarkable advance of scientific progress has not diminished that grim awareness of humanity, only exacerbated it—except, perhaps, in the minds of those who live in abject denial.

Chapter V

Culture of Denial

  A peasant farmer in Southeast Asia, planting seed in the spring and reaping harvest in the fall, is an apt witness of the seasonal gyrations that lead to the endless cycle of birth, death, and rebirth in the natural world. If the farmer seeks further answers, he discovers that birth and death are inextricably tied together in the entire natural order sustaining our planet. Life is a gift but it is not an infinite gift; it has a terminal point. It is imperative that we and the farmer understand this. Geological upheavals, wind, fire, water, and other natural phenomena, often destructive to fragile and embodied living things, are also vitally necessary for the organic life-and-death cycle of planet Earth. Without the uplifting of Earth's geological plates, sometimes accompanied by earthquakes and tsunamis, there would be no land above the sea. Contrastingly, Earth's celestial satellite, the moon, lacks atmosphere, seasonal change, wind, fire and, until recently, was thought to have no water. Currently, there is no indication of life. It is a silent orbiting mass.

  So long as we and our world are living, death is our inveterate companion, although I am told by my philosopher/scientist friend Holmes Rolston that "micro organisms just split in half and neither half has to die—they might get eaten or starve, but aging and death are not in their life process."[1] However, we human beings who have the capacity to contemplate our own deaths must come to terms with our own personal finiteness and that of our family, friends, and fellow travelers on this planet.

  If we are to remain healthy in mind and spirit, it is necessary that we become reconciled to the indisputable fact of death while, at the same time, seeking to avoid morbidity or denial in the process. Our occasional journeys through the clinical netherworld and at the bedsides of family and friends are among the events in life which present us with life's greatest tests and its inevitable conclusion. The ancient Hebrew psalmist laments, "The days of our years are threescore years and ten; and, if by reason of strength they be fourscore years, yet is their strength labor and sorrow; for it is soon cut off, and we fly away."[2] As previously mentioned, Christian scripture suggests that a sparrow cannot "fall on the ground without your Father."[3] Even with God's notice and presence, the sparrow still falls to the ground, a phenomenon that God does not intervene to prevent—it is the way of nature. Holmes Rolston reflects on the concurrence of natural science:

> In the end, any individual must die, by accident or by internal collapse, and here the death of earlier creatures makes room for later ones, room to live and, in time, to evolve. If nothing much had ever died, nothing much could have ever lived. Just as the individual overtakes, assimilates to itself, and discards its resource materials, so the evolutionary wave is propagated onward, using and sacrificing particulate individuals, which are employed in, but readily abandoned to, the larger currents of life. Thus the prolife evolution both overleaps death and seems impossible without it.[4]

Two decades ago, having been in contemplation about the likelihood of my own physical demise and death, I telephoned Luke Skelly, R.N., at that time the executive director of the Tennessee Donor Services. When he answered, I inquired, "Luke, if I die, what is the process for a complete donation of my body parts—tissue, organs, eyes, everything?" Immediately, he countered, "What do you mean if?"

Of course I got the point. It was not a question of "if" I die, but rather of "when." Having been professionally chastened by a friend, I realized that I was not unlike most other persons. We humans tend to view death subliminally or suppressively, as something that presents to others but not to ourselves, at least not right away. It was shortly after that when I made the first call to Vanderbilt University School of Medicine to inquire about anatomical gifts.

Anglican clergyman Jonathan Swift near the end of his life suffered significant mental and physical distress. However, earlier in his 1731 treatise, *Thoughts on Religion,* Swift commented reassuringly in words of comfort to others: "It is impossible that anything so natural, so necessary, and so universal as death, should ever have been designed as an evil to mankind."[5] If that be true, we ask, why do human beings innately have a tendency to deny death as it approaches, or when it occurs? In the netherworld experience at the bedside, it is more than likely that often it is this denial syndrome that affects our capacity to accept the reality of the unfolding drama or to make reasonable decisions concerning the moment of truth.

Ernest Becker provides perspective on this psychological phenomenon in his book, *The Denial of Death*. "The main thesis, [is that] . . . the idea of death, the fear of it, haunts the human animal like nothing else; it is a mainspring of human activity—activity designed largely to avoid the fatality of death, to overcome it by denying in some way that it is the final destiny for man."[6] In that regard, Becker continues in his book, "Freud discovered that each of us repeats the tragedy of the mythical Greek Narcissus: We are hopelessly absorbed with ourselves."[7] Perhaps the Albert Schweitzers and Mother Teresas of the world are exceptions to the blanket perception of Becker concerning the self-obsession of human beings, but I believe that it is applicable to the vast majority of us.

Even though my purpose in calling the donor service was to make casual preparation for the eventuality of my death, the subtle self-suggestion was that it may not happen—but if it did, it was not imminent. With similar reflection and disavowal, the vast majority of us human beings tend to put out of mind or to put off the process of handling wills and instructions relative to property, health-care decisions, or other important matters related to dying.

Children, youth, and young adults certainly do not dwell on the prospect that one day they will die, and rightly so. Such preoccupation on the part of the young would be construed as abnormal psychological dynamic, even though many of the cases considered in this book involve relatively young persons. As we mature in age, however, awareness of the possibility or probability of our own death is stimulated by natural events, illnesses, and aging occurring in the lives of each of us. When this happens, though, we more than likely push these thoughts down into the recesses of our subconscious minds and, when our children and youth inquire about death, we often are not prepared to deal adequately with their questions.

Consistent with beautiful natural philosophy, Miska Miles, a generation or two ago, wrote a lovely children's story that describes the life of a young Navajo Indian girl living in an adobe hut in the desert of the western United States with her mother, father, and grandmother.[8] One day, observing her grandmother weaving a rug, little Annie overheard the aged woman's remark, "When the rug is finished, I will die." Visibly upset, Annie went to bed that night with the words still in her mind. The next morning, when the family awakened, it was discovered that part of the woven yarn in the rug had been pulled out mysteriously during the night. After several more days of weaving and each subsequent morning finding the new portion removed, the grandmother realized that Annie surreptitiously had been unraveling the rug in hope that she would forestall the death of one whom she loved. A trip into the desert by grandmother and granddaughter, observing and discussing the birth, death, and rebirth cycle of the plants and animals, brought understanding and acceptance to the young heart and mind of Annie. This story by Miles, along with similar ones, is a wonderful teaching tool that has been adapted to preschool and early elementary curricula in various parts of the country to enrich children on the understanding and acceptance of death as a realistic and natural facet of life.

In similar sociologically naïve fashion as that of Annie, many in our contemporary culture have presented death and dying as an issue that is not being confronted as forthrightly as it should be. The subject, in its public and more violent form, is widely spread throughout our daily newspapers and blares forth in living color on our television screens. Nevertheless, there appears to be a psychological avoidance of death in its more personal and natural sense.

The famous botanist, Scottish-born John Muir, came with his family to America in 1849 when he was eleven years old. Immediately following the Civil War, he made enormous contributions in hands-on explorations, research, writings, and conversations relative to nature and the environment of planet Earth. In 1892, he founded the Sierra Club. His views on death, similar to those of Miles, are noteworthy:

> On no subject are our ideas more warped and pitiable than on death. Instead of the sympathy, the friendly

union, of life and death so apparent in Nature, we are taught that death is an accident. . . . But let children walk with Nature, let them see the beautiful blendings and communions of death and life, their joyous inseparable unity, as taught in woods and meadows, plains and mountains and streams of our blessed star, and they will learn that death is stingless indeed, and as beautiful as life, and that the grave has no victory. All is divine harmony.[9]

Even so, we should be intrigued by the fact that little has changed in human death culture for thousands of years. Furthermore, history supports the contention that the denial of death is endemic to human nature. The funeral practices of the Sumerian, Egyptian, and other ancient cultures confirm Becker's premise. Historians have advised us that the pyramids were not for the public activities of government and community (or mere architectural displays) but rather for religious purposes, designed to be the burial vaults for the self-serving kings and queens of Egypt, like Rameses, Tutenkhamon, Akenaten, and his wife Nefertiti.

"Apparently," says historian Will Durant, "the Pharaoh believed, like any other commoner among his people, that every living body was inhabited by a double, or Ka, which need not die with the breath; and that the Ka would survive all the more completely if the flesh were preserved against hunger, violence, and decay."[10] That clarifies why the pyramids were so huge. They had to be large enough to contain a ruler's wives, slaves, and elite guards, apparently most of whom were buried alive along with his expired, but specially prepared, body. The unfortunate attendants were considered necessities, along with the animals and various stores, for the continuing journey of the entourage in support of the one who has entered a *different* phase of life.

Jessica Mitford, along with others a generation ago, wrote of the extent to which a culture will go, not only in avoiding the reality of death but also in paying extravagantly for that avoidance. In her best-seller book, *The American Way of Death,* she described modern burial techniques which, in a relative sense, rival the ancient Egyptian monarchs with their lavishly appointed tombs:

> The emphasis is on the same desirable qualities that we have all been schooled to look for in our daily search for excellence: comfort, durability, beauty, craftsmanship. So that . . . solid flesh might not melt, we are offered solid copper—a quality casket which offers superb value to the client seeking long-lasting protection, or the Colonial Classic Beauty—18 gauge lead coated steel, seamless top, lap jointed welded body construction. Some are equipped with foam rubber, some with innerspring mattresses. Elgin offers the revolutionary Perfect Posture bed.[11]

Mitford initiated a revision of the book in the 1990s, and it was published two years after her own death in 1996. Such books document modern-day practices of the funeral industry, rituals that give impetus to the already existing cultural penchant for denying death or seeking to forestall it in the clinical setting and at the funeral parlor! My own thirty-six-year pastoral ministry experience and eighteen-year clinical ethics career confirm much of what she describes in her book.

While functioning as a pastor, I found that mortuary businesses, in the main, offer extremely helpful, sympathetic, and caring services to families in moments of sadness and grief. Several owners, managers, and their personnel have been among my very best colleagues through the years. Some of these persons have been extremely kind and generous in offering assistance in time of special need, when there have been deaths requiring services rendered at sharply reduced costs and, in several cases, at no cost at all. Having said that, I must admit that I have experienced with other servers some unusual circumstances and have witnessed extraordinary practices that only exacerbate the denial of death and its proliferating costs.

In its October 2009 news letter, AARP reported to its members, "According to the National Funeral Directors Association, the average cost of a regular adult funeral in 2006 was $7, 323, up 45 percent since 2001." Furthermore, the report states, "That figure does not include a cemetery plot, burial, a grave marker, flowers or other items that can add thousands of dollars to the average bill."[12]

In valiant efforts to suggest continuity and permanence, those who manufacture and sell funeral equipment and services oftentimes make exorbitant claims as to the eternal qualities of their burial hardware. I would argue that very expensive waterproof and airtight coffins, placed within very expensive waterproof and airtight vaults, only serve to accentuate the ambiguity of modern culture's succumbing to its superstitious primal instincts. Apparently many still believe, if only sentimentally, that one's "double" or "Ka" continues to exist in that body. The emphasis is upon preserving the body, shielding it from the elements and assuring that it will, physically at least, "rest in peace." For example, at the casket selection, one mortician said to a family in my presence, "Your loved one will be protected for eternity." I responded quizzically, "For eternity?" With a pained look, he responded, "Well, maybe not for eternity, but at least for a long, long time."

In stark contrast, some still raise the question, "Whatever happened to the old pine box?" Seemingly respondent to that question, one news source reported on the death and funeral arrangements of Ruth Graham, the wife of evangelist Dr. Billy Graham, in Montreat, N. C. near Asheville. "Reflecting her simple tastes, a casket built of plywood carried Ruth Bell Graham through the streets of her mountainside home in the Blue Ridge on Saturday [June 16, 2007]."[13] The Graham family perspective on death and interment is one that should be understood, appreciated, and emulated by others in our society. Another source reported also:

> Billy Graham, like his wife, will be buried in a birch plywood coffin built by inmates at Louisiana State penitentiary in Angola, La. The Graham's son Franklin made the request after seeing the coffins on a visit to the Angola prison and being struck by their simplicity, according to a statement from the Billy Graham Evangelistic Association. The coffins cost $215 each.[14]

Perhaps the death denial attitudes mentioned earlier explain the sign that I often see on the side of tractor trailer trucks on the interstate highways of the southeast. They transport coffins from a manufacturer to be distributed among funeral homes in the region.

The identifying company logo is alongside large letters that affirm: "Committed to the Dignity of Life." My view is that they do not have a primary commitment to life at all. On the contrary, they are committed to death and for some reason choose not to acknowledge it. Why not a "commitment to the dignity of death?" That is what coffins are really about. After all, this is a casket company dedicated to the manufacture of acceptable burial containers for dead bodies. On the right rear door of the truck transporting caskets, there is a final, spiritually insolent declaration for persons of faith to ponder: "Heaven can wait!"

Giving thanks for and memorializing the life of any human being, however, is an honorable endeavor. On the positive side again, funeral homes provide many worthwhile services for families at the death of a loved one. Respect for the dead and respect for their bodies, for closure in whatever state or form, should remain a critically important part of the grief associated with the loss of anyone—but not at the expense of sublimating or obscuring the fact that physical death is imminent or has occurred—the ultimate outcome of having been born into a world fraught with warfare, disease, and accidents. The clinical netherworld is the pervasive environment for experiencing the cultural phenomenon of the denial of death. Beyond its remarkably positive value, the advent of medical technology has exacerbated the penchant for disbelief that life's final days or hours have come for one's self or loved ones.

Dr. Holmes Rolston has argued in behalf of the necessity of the death process in the natural life of the planet, including that of homo sapiens and other animals. Becker appears to be supportive of that argument, when he concludes: "Manipulative, utopian science, by deadening human sensitivity, would also deprive men of the heroic, in their urge to victory. And we know that in some way this falsifies our struggle by emptying us, by preventing us from incorporating the maximum of experience."[15] Thus, I propose, contemporary clinical conditions are emerging to enhance the human being's inane susceptibility to the "technological delusion."

Chapter VI

Technological Delusions

The use of respirators, feeding tubes, and imaging procedures proliferated during the last half of the twentieth century and were merged with antibiotics and other medications. These unions produced a variety of new medical advances and procedures, which theretofore were not possible. Coinciding with worldwide improvements in sanitation and access to clean water and air, these medical breakthroughs have dramatically extended the parameters of life and forestalled death in many parts of the world. Medical developments are occurring at a dramatic pace. Expectations are at a new high, and we are rightly encouraged to persevere and not to give up easily when beset with accidents, illness, or aging. At the same time thousands of patients are sustained in horribly debilitated states for significant periods of time, subjected to procedures that have no medical benefit—procedures that become delusive and only add to the grief experienced by their families as well as to the spiraling clinical costs of health-care delivery.

It was such concerns that precipitated the recent attempt of some United States congressional leaders to ensure that vital conversations in the patient/physician relationship on living wills and durable powers of attorney for health care be maintained and that appropriate end-of-life issues be addressed in any new health-care legislation. A well-informed public hopefully will eschew efforts of partisan groups to diverge from the truth concerning such advance directives and who attach to them nebulous phrases like "death panels," in efforts to politicize needed reform in the health-care industry. On the positive side, it was also such concerns which precipitated an article by nationally syndicated columnist Ellen Goodman with the title, "Denial Continues to Drive High End-of-life Costs." Reinforcing our argument in the preceding chapter, in fact, Ms. Goodman wrote, "Today, more than one-fourth of Medicare dollars are spent in the last year of life. Most people want to die "peacefully" at home, but 80 percent die in hospitals. So, much of our money goes to the kind of death we don't want."[1]

Technology, combined with hubris resulting from scientific accomplishments, serves to magnify the subliminal myth that there are no natural limitations on life. We applaud those scientists already mentioned and others who continue to achieve heroic levels of research by raising the bar higher and still higher. But there is a recurring danger that our society will succumb to the prideful humanistic delusion that man is the measure of all things. Therefore, as scientists stretch the aging process and prolong impaired life, it is vital that we question whether or not physicians in the clinical settings should do everything they have the capacity to do, or that society insists that they do.

Among those initially raising such questions was Richard Lamm, former governor of Colorado. "The aging have a duty to die," exclaimed the governor twenty-five years ago in addressing his state's Health Lawyer's Association. Lamm's comments, taken by many out of the context of a more complete explanation, sent an alarming message to aging people in particular and a shiver down the spine of the public at large. Older citizens, who are often made to feel useless anyway, got the impression that contemporary society wanted to dispose of them, quietly, if possible. Outrage was expressed not only by the elderly but by those who care for them in private homes, hospitals, rehab centers, assisted living facilities, and nursing homes throughout the country. "Like leaves which fall off a tree forming the humus in which other plants can grow, we've got a duty to die and get out of the way with all of our machines and artificial hearts, so that our kids can build a reasonable life."[2] Lamm was using metaphors similar to the biological analogies on the necessity of death prescribed by fellow Coloradoan Holmes Rolston in the previous chapter, from his book *Science and Religion.* [3]

A careful examination of Governor Lamm's remarks, however, made it clear that his concerns were not slanted toward the aging alone. He was taking to task an unbridled scientific establishment and a society beginning to focus on technology as a classic panacea in the midst of a death-denying culture. He and others were questioning those health-care professionals who espouse the principles of medical vitalism, views which suggest that if physicians have the capacity to keep persons alive, even in conditions worse than death, then they are professionally and vocationally obligated to do so. Many of us in this country, along with Governor Lamm, question such flawed medical opinion and similarly misleading religious sentiment that espouses a religious vitalism. Over the last decade and a half, public conversations have periodically dredged up Lamm's comments from the past, according to sources at *The New York Times*: "In a letter dated Oct. 8, 1993, Mr. Lamm provided excerpts from the 1984 speech, in which he spoke philosophically about the terminally ill of any age, about the extraordinary coast of high-technology medicine and about the ability of medical science to stave off death far beyond considerations of quality of life."[4]

Aging persons themselves are anxious and somewhat frightened about the prospects of being placed on respirators and feeding tubes to be left with multi-system failure or in vegetative states. One elderly person some years ago said to me while on a pastoral visit, "I am not afraid to die. I *am* afraid of the long drawn-out procedure of dying that new medicine and new machines have made possible." Then she added, "I am concerned for myself being clinically oppressed, but also for my children who may have to make the hard decisions about withholding treatment."

It was such concerns that led physician Eric Cassell to devote the last chapter of his book, *The Healer's Art,* to what he described as "Overcoming the Fear of Death." He muses about the revered physician, William Osler, "Who once wrote that he could hardly remember a dying patient who was afraid of death." "That, too," Cassell observes, "has been my experience."[5] The experience of these two great physicians may be rebuttals of at least part of Becker's thesis that the "denial" of death springs from the "fear" of death. Therefore, Cassell concludes: "The sick deal with the concrete—pain, nausea, thirst, weakness, the fear that they won't be able 'to take it,' and so on. Those are the things that form the fears of the dying, and with good reason. They do not constitute the fear of death but rather the messy details and the burdens of dying."[6]

Additionally, there are concerns among and in behalf of the thousands of aging and disease-ridden patients being subjected to the "revolving door" syndrome in the last several days or weeks of their lives mentioned by Dr. Martenson in chapter III of this manuscript relative to a *New York Times* article. Often, the unfortunates are shuttled from home to hospital to nursing facility and then back again in a continuing cycle, invariably ending in death. Such patients frequently receive heroic treatments that beg the question on quality of life. Many patients are routinely subjected to burdensome surgical procedures and medical treatments that dramatically outweigh the benefits, usually at the insistence of well-meaning family members who are expecting the latest miracle. Leaning on prayer and enamored with technology, they arm themselves with the maxim, "One should never lose hope." Any thoughts or suggestions that they have abandoned their loved ones are summarily rejected. Surrounded by multiple technologies and medical possibilities, they find it difficult to separate hope from false hope. It is false hope that leads to denial. But the family requests are simple and straight-forward: "Do everything you can; we don't want to lose Mom!"

One example of technological delusion is the request for cardio-respiratory-resuscitation (CPR) attempted in the hospital as a response to unexpected cardiac arrest in critically ill patients. Families assume that if clinicians can only restore heart function and respiration, then there is hope for the renewing of a loved one, regardless of the negative medical indications. When a treatment plan for a terminally ill patient is discussed with family or surrogate, often there is the enjoinder: "We *do* want resuscitation in the event of cardiac arrest!" That is natural response, given the recent hype in this country relative to widespread public education and often positive usage of chest compression and, lately, the accessibility of portable defibrillators. It may sound odd to the layperson, but these procedures have a greater percentage of positive results outside the hospital, because they are usually administered to a person who has been in relatively good health up to the point of a sudden cardio-pulmonary episode or other crisis leading to sudden loss of breathing. However, resuscitation efforts with aging persons, or others of any age experiencing terminal illness in the hospital, are seldom successful. Most clinicians know CPR to be a brutal procedure that breaks ribs and breast bones of fragile patients and bears with it an extremely high clinical failure rate.

Such a negative statistic is not because of advanced age itself, but rather that the patient is in intensive care due to complex disease or multi-system end-of-life failures. One group of physicians writing in the *New England Journal of Medicine* concludes, "However, our findings suggest that age does not affect the prognosis for survival after resuscitation. . . . What determines prognosis is the underlying disease, not the year of birth."[7] In the *Journal of The American*

Medical Association, a similar judgment is succinctly offered, "Age alone independently determines neither survival nor quality of life after resuscitation."[8] When dire conditions have significantly compromised the patient, a grim outcome for CPR is essentially assured. Thus, orders in the patient's chart, Do Not Resuscitate, are important considerations for most terminally ill patients. These orders are written by the physician in consultation with the patient's family. They are critically important for family or surrogate understanding and acceptance. Some hospitals make this even more specific and call the non-procedure a DNAR (do not attempt resuscitation).

If resuscitation is facilitated with patients already in multi-system failure, the process invariably falls short and the patient dies anyway, or worse, the hapless patient is left in a permanent coma. Physicians, who know better, are often coerced by family members or surrogates who object when the issue of writing a Do Not Resuscitate order is posed. Sometimes it is easier for the physician not to write the order than it is to engage in time-consuming hassle or else be threatened with a malpractice suit by an anxious and overly demanding surrogate. Many times families want everything done that can be done, often resulting in procedures that are futile.

Thus, to do more is often worse than doing less when laypersons practice medicine and when physicians at times wittingly allow them to do it. The overriding question in doing any medical procedure is, "What is the perceived benefit to the patient?" If the answer is that there is little or no benefit, still another question should be asked, "Then why are we doing this procedure?" Physicians and hospitals have a moral and legal obligation not to deliver costly services that are unnecessary or reasonably non-beneficial. CPR is one such procedure that often falls short in the clinical setting. The American Medical Association and its Council On Ethical and Judicial Affairs states, "Physicians are not ethically obligated to deliver care that, in their best judgment will not have a reasonable chance of benefiting their patients. Patients should not be given treatments simply because they demand them."[9]

Closely associated with resuscitation efforts is the use of the respirator. If cardio-respiratory function is artificially induced, then continuation of that function often depends on an artificially supplied technology. From birth until death, when an animal of any species is deprived of life-sustaining oxygen carried by the bloodstream to all parts of the body, atrophy and death are imminent. The value of oxygen for human life was never so poignantly demonstrated as the day when I was called to give spiritual support at the bedside of a young woman who had just delivered a beautiful son—stillborn! The lifeless baby was lying on a table in the room when I entered. As I gazed down at the perfectly formed infant, I expected him at any moment to begin crying, but he never did. The placenta had separated from the wall of the uterus while the baby was still in the birth canal. In the process of being born, the baby tragically suffocated from the lack of oxygen in the blood being channeled through the placenta from the mother to her newborn.

So, if birth occurs, the breathing capacity of the body (inhalation of oxygen and exhalation of carbon dioxide) becomes a vital function in maintaining life. Some at the bedside may believe, as discussed in an earlier chapter, as long as there is a heartbeat, hope remains for the life of the loved one. Many assume also that when the natural heart fails and an artificial ventilator/respirator substitutes, hope abides—as long as the substitute remains in place. What is not understood is that in many situations having a heart beat, in and of itself, is medically misleading, as was discussed in an earlier chapter. Often it is not enough for survival. The fervent resistance to the removal of a respirator from a dying patient thus has to be considered within the contextual health of the brain and other vital centers of the body.

A third example of technologically induced delusion is the use of feeding and hydration tubes at the end of life. Nutrition and hydration, when utilized under medically appropriate circumstances, appear to be precious ingredients for the continuation of life, though they are not without risks. In a published article in 2005, Lisa Green wrote concerning the origin of feeding and hydration tubes:

> The ancient Egyptians used reeds and animal bladders to supply patients with a mix of wine, chicken broth, and raw eggs. . . . Over the centuries, attempts to feed people have included trying to give nutrition rectally, as the Egyptians and doctors for President James Garfield did. After Garfield was shot in 1881, he stayed alive for 79 days on a mix of beef broth and whiskey. In 1969, University of Pennsylvania doctors

made a huge leap forward by keeping a baby girl alive for nearly two years with intravenous nutrition.[10]

In the last quarter of the twentieth century, such tubes, inserted through the nose or into the stomach, initially were designed to give premature or incapacitated newborns the nutrition necessary to survive a medically compromised stage and then to move on, hopefully to a more stable and healthy life. Initially, it was not intended that a feeding tube be a procedure of clinical choice for the long-term care of individuals. The use of this technology and treatment gravitated upwards in the 1980s through the newly born infant, child, youth, and adult levels of illness to assist persons in a variety of clinically acute situations. Feeding tubes have no intrinsically curative value, but may offer substantive support and hope that a potential procedure or medication can effect an improvement in a patient suffering from failure to thrive, disease, or accidents. Thus, tube-feeding procedures were particularly welcomed for an interim purpose in situations where the benefits of treatment outweighed the burdens and there was hope of recovery.

However, the technology made its way into clinical cases that necessitated perpetual care, where the burdens of treatment significantly outweighed the benefits of treatment. In an article entitled "Feeding Tubes and IVs at the End of Life," R.N. Angela Morrow also makes the case that artificial intravenous feeding and hydration are not without risks. She asks the question, "Is artificial nutrition beneficial for the terminally ill patient?" Then she proceeds with some medical data which suggest that total parenteral nutrition, nasogastric feeding tubes, gastrostomy tubes, and intravenous hydration are fraught with risks and, often as not, fail "to increase the health or life expectancy of the patient."[11] Whether in persistent vegetative cases involving brain-damaged young adults or aging persons afflicted with end-stage Parkinson's, Alzheimer's, or other "advanced" dementias, the nature and value of tube feeding is therefore highly questionable. In most end-of-life situations tube feeding does not provide a cure or medical benefit.

Thus, I would argue that studies show that such technology often becomes a curse instead of a blessing, a millstone around the neck of the dying patient. Dr. Eric Raefsky, a Nashville clinical oncologist on the staff at Summit Medical Center, acceded to the request of the ethics committee that he provide a concise statement on use of feeding tubes in terminally ill cancer patients. He responded in part as follows:

> Since there is no scientific basis to support the use of intensive nutritional support in this setting, it is difficult to justify its use from a moral or ethical perspective. Again, patients with terminal cancer die from overwhelming cancer, not malnutrition. In fact, the whole issue of nourishment often causes denial and conflict between patients and loved ones. A poor appetite is often used as an excuse for the deterioration of a patient ('if only he would eat he would do better'), thereby preventing patients and a family dealing with the real issues of impending death and dying.

Clinically intractable persons, ordinarily family or friends of terminally ill patients, and some medical and many religious professionals, assume that it is inhumane to deprive persons of that which they believe to be essential to life itself. Beyond oxygen, the least one can do, they say, is to provide food and water. Viewing the respirator as an "extraordinary" medical treatment that may be withheld or withdrawn at the end of life, the Vatican driven Roman Catholic Church considers nutrition and hydration efforts as "ordinary" medical treatments that should be continued until the patient dies. Catholic moral theologian Daniel Maguire, and others in that faith tradition, disagree with this Vatican position as does this author, from within a Protestant tradition. These sustaining ingredients, so basic and vital to the health of normal human beings, are likely to be counterproductive and even burdensome to a person in the final stages of an illness. Fluids, in the form of nutrition and hydration, can create systemic stress within a failing body that has become naturally anorexic.

Howard Brody, et al, in a *New England Journal of Medicine* article affirmed some years ago, "Although there are numerous case reports and few controlled studies, the emerging consensus suggests that seriously ill or dying patients experience little if any discomfort on the withdrawal of tube feedings, parenteral nutrition, or intravenous hydration." Then they conclude, "Compelling case reports illustrate the high level of comfort and satisfaction among patients that may accompany dying after refusing nutrition and hydration, even in cases in which survival is prolonged."[12] In a near-death state, the person ordinarily has no sense of hunger and thirst, nor does the body itself crave or need nutrition and hydration. Essentially, the person in this state dies first, not of malnutrition but rather of dehydration, not an unpleasant death given the presence of the other disease factors leading to the demise in the first place.

    Some years ago, as a clinical ethicist, I participated on a panel with several others, a registered nurse, a chaplain, a certified social worker, and a physician. The one-hundred-plus attendees were gathered in a workshop for nursing home medical and nursing directors from across the state of Tennessee. Commenting on the need to rethink the use of feeding tubes in many end-of-life situations, I made the point that my physician friends tell me that death by dehydration is not an unpleasant death. On the contrary, that it is a merciful and sometimes preferred way to allow the natural death to occur when the end is imminent.

    Suddenly, a person on the back row stood up and shouted, "You are *not* a physician, and I *am*; I disagree with you!" Just as forcefully, a person to my right on the panel stood up and said to the physician on the back row, "I *am* a physician, and I disagree with you!" The panelist was Jack Moore, a medical doctor on the staff of Cookeville (Tennessee) General Hospital and medical director of a nursing home in that city. Gratefully, I sat down and let him continue speaking to those assembled. He went on to cite an epic of death and survival during the Second World War.

    Captain Eddie Rickenbacker, famous pilot in World Wars I and II, was on a mission with seven others, flying in a B-17 over the Pacific in 1942. Before reaching their destination, the eight airmen were forced to ditch the plane in the sea. Clinging to three rubber rafts tied together and with almost no supplies, they were at the mercy of the elements. What little food they had was soon gone along with a scant amount of fresh water a few days later. At one point, they bit-by-bit consumed the remains of a sea gull that had been captured after perching on the tiny rafts. On the fourteenth day, one of their companions succumbed to the ordeal. He was buried at sea. The remaining seven among their number survived for twenty-four days. All were subjected to exposure, dehydration, starvation, and were barely alive when found. They reported later that, with no perceived physical anguish, the person who died simply curled up, went to sleep, and did not awaken. If he had received just a bare amount of nutrition and water, the courageous airman perhaps would not have died, since there were no other medical anomalies involved. In his swift rebuttal, Dr. Jack Moore concluded, "Based on these data and numerous other similarly tragic episodes, scientists began to rewrite the medical textbooks on understanding this type of dying process and appropriate care for patients in the related final stages of life. Then, in the last quarter of the twentieth century we were led astray in treating those terminally ill from other causes, by the futile use of feeding and hydration tubes."

Thus, in recent decades, leading medical journals have been filled with articles questioning the use of ill-advised resuscitation and prolonged tube feeding/hydration efforts in situations that offer no medical benefit and where the dying process becomes a diagnosed reality. There is a proven better way to care for the terminally ill. Commensurately, physicians and nurses are becoming educated and skilled in the recognition and management of pain and discomfort. Often, the dying process is allowed to continue its natural course, framed by hospice-type care. The term *palliate*, to relieve or mitigate, is the moral linchpin that lies at the center of the humane, much less expensive clinical procedure leading to the natural death of a patient.

However, the fact that hospice care is significantly less expensive than technologically intensive treatment, cost is not, in and of itself, the conceptus that drives end-of-life decisions. I will argue that focus upon whether or not a treatment is beneficial to the patient, not the expense, determines the moral appropriateness or inappropriateness of a medical decision impacting terminal cases. If the medical procedure cannot offer an advantage to the patient, then it must be perceived as having no medical value. Not only are some procedures at the end of life of no value to the patient, they may be, in fact, further detrimental to the fragile well being of the dying patient and the patient's family. Why would anyone insist on continuing complex but useless medical procedures which categorically fall short of some of the perceived goals of medicine, that is, to improve patient mental or physical status, to effect a cure, to do no harm, and to do what is beneficial? At the outset of this book, Professor McKenzie made the point that ethics and morality have to do with the *good* of a person! In providing no *good* for the patient, I maintain that such medical treatment makes no ethical sense, that it creates a state of cultural and technological denial and, in the final analysis, is fiscally irresponsible and morally unjust.

Chapter VII

Quality of Life Pitted Against Sanctity of Life

Frau Meier and Sibyl

"To experience the death of a person is to acknowledge defeat," we were told by physicians in 1989 as we stood in the doorway of the critical intensive unit of the Augsburg Zentralkliniken, a major Bavarian hospital in the Federal Republic of Germany, immediately before the reunification, West and East. As if to augment the relevance of this clinical statement, we observed the moribund body and unresponsive mind of a tiny woman, stripped to the waist. Gastrointestinal feeding tube, central intravenous line, total parenteral nutrition bottles, and assorted monitoring tabs were attached to her nude upper body. A catheter protruded from her motionless torso and an attached bag dangled at the bedside, with a white sheet covering her lower extremities. Assisted cardio-respiratory function was evident, but she remained in a comatose state.

Suffering from the advanced stages of Addison's disease, the adrenal glands experienced acute failure, and the muscular structure had collapsed. Surgical and medical procedures at an earlier point produced no improvement in the downward spiral. Mucous membranes were critically involved with the end-stage crisis. Skin pigmentation had turned dark brown, almost black. Life was at its lowest stage. After discussing the medical indications and viewing the physical condition of the patient, one had to wonder why she had been maintained at that stage for more than ninety days on support systems. Nurses in the unit reported that they had queried the attending physicians about the untenable life support for this patient in multi-system failure for such an extensive period. They were told by the physicians, "You are reacting with feelings, and feelings alone are not adequate criteria for making medical decisions."

The Augsburg facility in 1989 was an impressive, recently constructed 1,400-bed tertiary care medical center. There was also an adjoining 250-bed children's clinic, and an 80-bed psychiatric building soon to be expanded to 250 beds. Apparent at every level was the very latest technologically advanced health-care delivery. "The goal of medicine in these facilities," another physician affirmed, "is to enable sick people to recover and to forestall death as long as possible." I have encountered physicians in the clinical setting in the United States who practice similarly aggressive medicine. Some were practicing medicine from a professionally forceful medical perspective with a mixture of fundamentalist religion. I do not know the underlying motivation of the German physician in declaring the goal for his medical practice.

Dr. Georg Dellbrugge, my Bavarian host, and I observed the woman lying with terribly compromised quality of life pitted against sanctity of life in the Medical Intensive Care Unit of this ultramodern hospital. We named her Frau Meier, the German equivalent of Jane Doe in America. There seemed to be in our minds, and those of the nurses at the bedside, an ethical dissonance, a moral incongruity, separating the second expressed goal of the physician from the first. Certainly, one of the first goals of medicine, universally, is "to enable sick people to recover." That is indisputable. The accompanying expressed goal of the Augsburg physician, "to forestall death as long as possible" may very well be morally repugnant when the possibility of restoring health to a patient is improbable—as with this case and similar ones observed in the United States. The Hippocratic principle, "First do no harm," is a major concern when the continuation of intensively delivered medicine over a long period of time appears to be nonproductive. As argued earlier, when the burdens of treatment outweigh the benefits, or appear to have no benefit at all, then one must seriously question the continued medical maintenance of the patient, which itself may be a harm to the patient and to the family, if there is one. We were not told whether Frau Meier had ever expressed her wishes for treatment or if there ever were a surrogate or family in consultation with the physicians treating her.

The spectacle of the diminutive woman lying on a bed of the intensive care unit in Augsburg in 1989 conjured up for me a mental image of Sibyl, a character in an epigraph in Petronius' *Satyricon* from the seventh century AD in Rome. That satire was shared by ethicist/attorney David Smith in a 1984 brain death symposium at Vanderbilt. Sibyl, a young Roman woman, asked the pagan gods for the gift of eternal life, a request which, in turn, was granted. A critical point, however, was that Sibyl did not simultaneously receive *eternal youth*! So, passing through the generations, she continued to live, growing older and older, shriveling up to become a tiny figure enclosed in a bottle at Cumae, one of the centers for pagan worship. An acolyte passed by, and seeing her hanging there, asked, "Sibyl, what do you wish?" She replied, "I wish to die."[1] Frau Meier, in Augsburg, was not hanging in a bottle, but therapeutic bottles were hanging all over *her*, hooked to lines protruding from her minute torso, which appeared to be pleading silently for relief.

As mentioned, the visit to Germany in 1989 occurred shortly before the collapse of the Berlin Wall and reunification of West and East. The West German public sector, as well as mainstream medical professionals in clinical settings, appeared to shun open discussion of complex end-of-life medical issues. Except for articles in professional journals and occasional symposia in major academic settings, there seemed to be little public interchange of ideas among the German people as a whole on the ethics of health-care delivery, especially at the end of life. Dr. George Hermann Dellbrugge, now retired, was Professor of Philosophy and Religion at Augustana Hoschule, in Neuendettelsau, Germany and a similar institution in Munich. He was a visiting professor of Medical Ethics in 1988 at the Vanderbilt University Center for Clinical and Research Ethics in Nashville. It was there, when I was Associate Director of the Center, that we met. Upon his return to Neuendettelsau in Bavaria, a small city almost midway between Munich and Nuremburg, he invited me to present a formal paper at university city academies in those two larger cities, where he taught as well. The issues pertained to clinical concerns at beginning and end of life. Professor Dellbrugge and I also participated in informal discussions on clinical medical ethics with very receptive medical, nursing, and chaplain staffs in seven hospitals in the cities of Augsburg, Munich, Nuremburg, Rummelsburg, and a perpetual care facility in Neuendettelsau, for persons with severe physical deprivations at birth.

A Lutheran hospital chaplain expressed concerns similar to those of the Augsburg nurses and several physicians when we met with him in the still larger 2000-bed Ludwig-Maximillian University Hospital in Munich. "This is the best place in the world to receive the latest surgical procedure and medical treatment," he lamented, "but it is not the best place to get healthy." The halls of this gigantic hospital extended horizontally over 200 meters at each of its 14 levels.

Pointing with great pride to the impressive surgical floor containing 36 operating rooms, the chief of surgery asserted proudly, "We see to it that no one dies in these units." The chagrined observation of another physician serving on a bone-marrow transplant team set things in perspective, however: "Surgery," he commented, almost apologetically, "is done much faster and more frequently than the healing—death and dying are simply passed on to other units."

He then stated flatly that German physicians, at that time, continued to practice medicine in what has been called "isolated dyads." As if to prove that point, still another physician in Munich told us, "Physicians feel very responsible for clinical treatment plans, and they make those decisions unilaterally in behalf of the patient" (the epitome of medical paternalism). Then he added, "I do what is best—I have the training to do what is best." No one doubted his training and ability, but the asymmetrical relationship between doctor and patient was remarkably evident. The patient had little or no input, with scant involvement in the decision-making process. One can only hope that such imbalance in the patient-physician relationship has undergone significant change since the visit to Germany twenty-one years ago.

Postal, e-mail and telephone conversations with my German philosopher/theologian friend George have indicated that change *is* occurring in the patient and physician relationship since the visit twenty years ago. Paternalism existing simultaneously in the United States, though not as pronounced, has likewise essentially moderated during a similar period of time. The moral and legal emphasis on the patient's right of autonomy and subsequent medical self-determination have brought symmetry to the patient-physician relationship in the United States, which now assumes a more negotiable mode.

The emphasis in that Munich hospital, as with Augsburg, was quite obviously upon perfection of surgical techniques and the use of technology and procedures to sustain life, with less emphasis on life's quality. Sanctity of life appeared to be an absolute value, which prevailed over all other considerations. It was as though "forestalling death, not acknowledging defeat, and doing what is best," using the words of the physicians, were ends in themselves. This was clearly medical vitalism of the first order, elements of which remain today in American practice of medicine and public perception as well. Such clinical forcefulness assumes almost absolute value, greater than that of the patient's best interest, the patient's right to be informed, and the patient's right to choose. Twenty years later in the United States, the broadly based public reaction to the Terri Schiavo persistent vegetative case is ample evidence that medical aggressiveness is still robust in the minds of some physicians and in the citizenry as a whole (See Ch. X. of this book).

The comments by health-care professionals took on additional relevance several days later in a Nuremburg university center. Professor Dellbrugge and I were presenting papers on "Beginning of Life—End of Life Issues." A medical doctor in the audience observed afterwards, "The German health-care system is trapped somewhere between Hitler and Hackethal." He went on to explain that Adolf Hitler represented the holocaust, the Nazi experimental atrocities and genocide in places like Auschwitz, Buchenwald, and Dachau. German medical doctors, along with political and military leaders, were placed on trial at Nuremburg following World War II. Out of twenty-three indicted physicians, sixteen were found guilty.[2] Biomedical research had been ordered by the ruthless Nazi hierarchy as a ruse to exterminate Jews throughout Europe, but also to eradicate the mentally ill, the intellectually retarded, and the physically disabled from the "master race" society. After the verdicts at Nuremberg, the American Military Tribunal adopted The Nuremburg Code, relative to medical experimentation on human beings. There were ten principles recommended. Excerpts of the first two principles are as follows:

> 1. The voluntary consent of the human subject is absolutely essential. This means that the person involved should have legal capacity to give consent; should be so situated as to be able to exercise free power of choice, without the intervention of any element of force, fraud, deceit, duress, over-reaching, or other ulterior form of constraint or coercion; and should have sufficient knowledge and comprehension of the elements of the subject matter involved as to enable him to make an understanding and enlightened decision.

2. The experiment should be such as to yield fruitful results for the good of society, unprocurable by other methods or means of study, and not random and unnecessary in nature.[3]

As a result of sensitivity to these abominations, Germany's physicians, along with those in the United States and elsewhere, were therefore practicing aggressively conservative medicine in the midst of burgeoning technology. Terminally ill patients were being placed in a techno-structured health-care delivery system in which hardly anyone was allowed to die easily or quickly. Many physicians withdrew life support only after applying every other possible treatment and procedure; none wanted to be called a Nazi! Similar unease, following the Nuremberg trials, spread worldwide and influenced medical research and medical practice almost universally.

In the 1980s, Julius Hackethal, on the other hand, was a contemporary German physician who thought that he had perfected a remarkably successful surgical cure for cancer. As it evolved, his clinical methodology was no more effective than the current norm, and he turned, in his disappointment, to the hospice care of terminally ill patients. Then, in 1984 Dr. Hackethal, in a manner similar to that of Dr. Jack Kevorkian's 1990s efforts in the United States, overzealously sought to dramatize what he truly perceived to be the most humane care for the dying. He videotaped the last moments of a patient to whom he had given a lethal injection, and he later presented the tape for public viewing in living color on West German television. This created a wave of revulsion on the part of health-care professionals and the lay public in that country. Thus, driven by the extremes of both Hitler and Hackethal, a dramatic counter movement embraced thorough-going sanctity-of-life perspectives.

Mainly, this clinical paranoia has partly delayed progress toward appropriate removal of futile life support systems in Germany. It exacerbated non-beneficial medical procedures for terminally ill patients as it has somewhat in the United States in response to Kevorkian. Whereas, in 1989 the German health-care system partly found itself trapped between Hitler and Hackethal, the recipient of health care, the patient, was imprisoned within historic social and political principles. The much-used phrase "alles in ordnung" (everything in order) presented the patient in a clinical setting reluctant to question authority. The authority was in the hands of the physician who made unilateral decisions.

There was relative public reticence to question medical science's aggressive use of advanced technology for which German scientists have a natural passion and inventiveness—and for which the world owes a great debt. Patient unwillingness to affirm the right to medical self-determination, or uncertainty about that right, apparently projected informed consent forms and living wills into the health-care system as somewhat symbolic guides for physicians. My impression was that of an environment in Germany with a limited concern for the issues of medical malpractice. It thus manifested itself in a far less litigious atmosphere than exists in the United States.

Furthermore, the same unwillingness and uncertainty projected a general lack of clinical and public dialogue concerning complex medical issues and patient rights in that country. On the other hand, it is a fact that litigation in the historic U.S. court cases has led to a more extensive discussion of these issues in the last quarter of a century, although a federal judge friend of mine in Nashville observed some years ago that these critical issues are best resolved at the bedside in the patient/family/physician relationship and should remain outside the courts, which are the places of last resort.

Essentially, the clinical ethics posture of many in the German Republic in 1989, as well as here in the United States, demonstrated a formidable blend of medical aggressiveness, sanctity of life, and technology. Medicine, universally, has espoused the principle that the state has a compelling duty to preserve life. Sanctity of life, on the other hand, is carried to its ultimate level in this triad; that is, all other values are superseded by the absolute value of human life. Medical aggressiveness expands the principle that patients should be kept alive in all possible circumstances and at all costs. This is precisely the scientific determinism that Governor Lamm of Colorado was railing against years ago in speaking to his state's health lawyers, specifically, the view that, "everything which can be done must be done."

Consistent with Governor Lamm's call for minute examination, even the U.S. Roman Catholic bishops, in giving guidance to their constituents, differ in part from the vitalist/sanctity/absolutist position. In their Ethical and Religious

Directives for Catholic Health Services, the Bishops state, at least at this point exclusive of nutrition and hydration tubes:

> We have a duty to preserve our life and to use it for the glory of God, but the duty to preserve life is not absolute, for we may reject life-prolonging procedures that are insufficiently beneficial or excessively burdensome. Suicide and euthanasia are never morally acceptable options.[4]

> The determination of death should be made by the physician or competent medical authority in accordance with responsible and commonly accepted scientific criteria.[5]

Similarly, the General Assembly of the Presbyterian Church U.S, in 1981 counseled its members through an officially adopted report presented its Counsel on Theology and Culture:

> Finally, the limit on the ability of human life to bear pain and suffering needs to be noted. There is a point at which pain and suffering can debilitate life beyond recognition. If pain and suffering are of a constancy and intensity which make relatedness to others impossible; and if there is no reasonable prospect for relief that would make such relief actual—there arises the question of whether preservation of life is a binding obligation. In such a situation it may be a more adequate avoidance of harm and even of promoting well-being, to allow death to occur.[6]

The cases of Karen Ann Quinlan, Nancy Cruzan, Terri Schiavo, Paul Brophy, Jane Doe, and Nancy Gamble in subsequent chapters offer examples of sanctity of life pitted against quality of life. The earlier of those tragic episodes led philosopher Daniel Callahan to argue that "technology had co-opted the sanctity of life principle." Dr. Callahan places his finger on the vital nerve center of this issue: "Medical science is very clever in making us feel guilty about accepting the end of human life; in the hubris, it has led us to think of death as a curable condition, or at least indefinitely postponable."[7]

As stated earlier and expanded here, physician Edmund D. Pelligrino was among those in the medical profession acknowledging the need for and calling for the clinical participation of philosophers such as Richard Zaner, Dan Callahan, Robert Veatch and others, who look with critical analysis and apply collective values to strategically important human endeavors, none more important than within the health-care institution. Dr. Pelligrino wrote three decades ago:

> The terms value and purpose are beginning to appear for the first time as respectable subjects for clinical inquiry. With the effective means modern science provides, the physician must determine whether or not he should use the techniques he possesses for whom, for what purpose, and according to what value system. The prolongation of life, abortion, genetic counseling, dangerous operative and diagnostic procedures—all involve an intersection of the values of the patient, society, and the physician. . . . Moreover, the sciences are too susceptible to seductions of the 'technological imperative' to be safe guides through such intricacies.[8]

The pathetic stories of Frau Meier and Sibyl clearly present the issue of quality of life pitted against sanctity of life. As posited earlier, both were in states worse than death. It is one matter to hang on to hope, as long as it offers a reasonable chance of recovery or a return to a quality of life that is bearable. It is another thing to descend to the level of incurable morbidity of a Frau Meier or to the state of inescapable pathos of a satiric Sibyl. It is therefore critical that there be those at the bedside who continually pose the question—whether they be professional or nonprofessional: "What is the value and purpose of, and prognosis for, this procedure?"

Mary Northern

The term *quality of life* has somewhat of an elusive and uncertain characteristic. I would argue that quality of life, like beauty, is in the eye of the beholder. Sanctity of life, similarly, is limited by its finiteness and therefore is not itself an absolute value. It is imperative, therefore, that the patient who has a clear mental capacity, with a competency to choose, must be the ultimate "decider" on treatment or non-treatment issues affecting one's self. The case of Mary Northern, because of its ambiguous ingredient, is worthy of our review.

On a cold January day in 1978, a seventy-two year old Nashvillian was warming herself before an open free-standing grill in a fireplace. Inadvertently, she knocked the device over, spilling the hot coals onto her ankles and feet. Neighbors, noticing the smoke emanating from the house, called police. Twice the authorities came to her door and twice she turned them away. A third time they came back and, against her will, forcibly removed her from her home. Placing her in the police car, the officers took her to the Metropolitan Nashville General Hospital. There, she was given medical treatment, which likewise was delivered against her will.

After several days in the medical center, a serious infection developed in Ms. Northern's feet, and she was informed by the physicians that it might be necessary to amputate them. Though obviously eccentric, Mary Northern was nevertheless quite an intelligent homeowner who had simply chosen to live to herself, a recluse, apart from her neighbors and society in general. She refused to grant permission for the feet to be excised, even when physicians advised her repeatedly that her intransigence could lead to her death. Subsequently, the Tennessee Department of Human Services and the courts became involved. After ten days a Chancery Court judge appointed a young Nashville Attorney, Carol McCoy, as guardian ad litem.[9]

By this time, gangrene had developed in both feet, and the physicians kept warning that the situation was grave. Once more the courts became involved, and attorney McCoy, convinced that Mary Northern was of sound mind, filed a brief requesting that forced amputation be denied. The attorney was adamant that Ms. Northern had counted the cost of refusing amputation. She believed that, for Mary Northern, it was a quality-of-life issue; she simply did not want to live without her feet. After a relatively short hearing, the judge ruled that since the medical situation was deteriorating and apparently was life threatening, both feet should be removed within twenty-four hours.

Attorney McCoy then asked the court's permission to allow a psychiatrist to examine Miss Northern as to her competency to refuse consent (i.e., to refuse treatment). The right of refusal was hers by law if she were found to be of sound mind. The patient was examined by a psychiatrist whose approach was through a relatively unique set of questions that placed Mary Northern in a "Catch 22" situation. His questions were based on the premise that if she would agree that her situation was serious and that the amputation should proceed, then he would declare her to be competent. On the other hand, if she did not agree that her feet should be removed, then he would opine that she was incompetent. In my opinion this is a classic example of logically "begging the question."

However, upon that line of reasoning and psychological examination, the judge ruled that the amputation should proceed on the basis of what is called "selective incompetence"—a sort of temporary inability to make sound judgments, at least on this particular issue. During this interim period, pneumonia developed. Mary Northern, struggling with the added medical problem along with the gangrenous condition of her feet, still refused to give permission for the surgery. Unwilling to have her feet amputated, the determined patient and her equally determined legal advocate were granted an appeal to a higher court. Over several days, appellate court judges went to the hospital to question the patient. She was adamant. If she were going to die, it was her wish that she would do so with feet intact.

The appeals court, in turn, upheld the lower court's ruling of "selective incompetence." She was deemed competent in other matters related to her well-being, but in this particular medical situation Mary Northern was declared incompetent to make a decision in her own behalf. Subsequently, Attorney McCoy filed further appeals.

In the meantime, Mary Northern successfully waged a battle against two life-threatening anomalies, pneumonia and gangrene. Ironically, having begun in January of 1979 the fight to choose her own destiny, she was still maintaining her desire and right to refuse amputation, when she died of a heart attack. During the hospitalization, blood clotting developed as a result of the extensive use of antibiotics to combat the pneumonia and gangrene. Her four month legal struggle ended when she died on May 15, with her case review pending before the State of Tennessee Supreme Court. At Miss Northern's death, the case was dismissed without a judgment of the court.

The facts of this unusual case not only pit quality of life against sanctity of life but should make one aware of the delicate and sometimes vague balance required in making appropriate and humane decisions—along with the equally vague question of determining competency in clinical and courtroom settings. In an article entitled "The Many Faces of Competency," James Drane writes, "As long as a patient does or says nothing strange and acquiesces to treatment by the medical profession, questions of competency do not arise."[10]

Mary Northern's competency, I would argue, was *suspect* the moment she ordered the policemen away from her door. Related questions continued throughout her hospital odyssey when she consistently refused treatment which, in the best medical professional opinion, would save her life. Retrospectively, in these pages, I cannot judge Mary Northern's capacity to make appropriate decisions; I can only cite the case as a unique quality-of-life issue to be faced. However, I agree with James F. Drane's conclusion that in all cases, "More careful evaluation is then called for before a final determination of competency is made."[11] The line between the state's overriding responsibility to uphold and to protect the sanctity of life and the right to individual self-determination of life's quality is a thin one indeed. However, it is my opinion, as has been one of the thesis in this book, that when quality of life is pitted against sanctity of life, it is the right of the competent adult human being to determine what shall happen to one's own body. I submit, as well, that eccentricity and mental incapacity to decide are not synonymous.

Part Two

We have been advancing a premise that human life, though often constricted by disease and impairments and limited by death, is a value of first order, and that one's right to personal choice in health-care decision making is a matter of priority as well. The presentations, questions, and cases that follow, are intended to add to these discussions from the author's experience and perspective on withholding and withdrawing care. The President's Commission for the Study of Ethical problems in Medicine and Biomedical and Behavioral Research in 1981 recommended the Determination of Death Act, which subsequently has been ratified by all fifty of the United States of America:

> An individual who has sustained either (1) irreversible cessation of circulatory and respiratory functions, or (2) irreversible cessation of all functions of the entire brain, including the brain stem, is dead. A determination of death must be made in accordance with accepted medical standards.

This definition pertains to death by whole-brain criteria and is applicable to the case of Taylor Coleman, which follows immediately. Commensurately, Philosopher Richard Zaner has stated: "The new technologies now make it possible for us to sustain bodies which will never again embody a conscious person."[1] His reference here is acknowledgement of the persistent vegetative state wherein human bodies are maintained for indeterminable periods of time in horribly debilitated states. This tragic medical anomaly caused by a physical insult to the neo-cortex results in the loss of higher brain function and manifests itself in "partial brain death," in contrast with whole brain criteria.

Such cases are those of non-sentient Karen Ann Quinlan, Paul Brophy, Nancy Cruzan, and Terri Schiavo, which present sequentially, after the one of Taylor Coleman. Thus, argument will be made in support of those who advance the need for an additional determination of death based on neocortical criteria and a plea by

Attorney/Ethicist David Smith and many others for the adoption of a related definition of neocortical death. The lack of such a definition, in my view, supports arguments which decry the pervasive denial of justice at the end of life.

Chapter VIII
Whole-Brain Death

Taylor Coleman

On Friday evening, July 7, 1972, A.J. and Shirley Coleman were entertaining house guests in their gracious home in Decatur, Alabama. The reunited friends were lightheartedly discussing plans for their high school reunion the next day. Within hours, however, they began a descent into the harsh realm of the netherworld. The prominent attorney and his wife were also awaiting the arrival of their seventeen-year-old son Taylor. He was expected home that evening, having attended a week-long church youth conference at Camp Nacome near Centerville, Tennessee. Though the conference officially ended the next morning, an earlier ride with a local pastor had been arranged. That schedule offered Taylor an adequate night's rest before taking his college SAT test on that July 8, Saturday at 9:00 a.m. Stunning 6-foot-3-inch, 190-pound teenager Taylor Coleman was a rising high school senior.

At midnight, still with no Taylor and no telephone calls, the concerned parents were becoming anxious. The presence of their house guests made the slowly passing time a bit easier until the two couples retired for the night. When the phone did ring about 2:30 a.m., their utmost fears were harshly realized. An automobile accident occurred shortly after midnight on a dark two-lane highway near Columbia, Tennessee. Taylor Coleman canceled his earlier departure on Friday to travel home with two teen-age friends from nearby Huntsville who were leaving later in the evening. Seventeen-year-old John A. Scoble, Jr., was driving the car with another teenage friend in the right front seat. After reflecting with the others on the highpoints of the previous five days, Taylor fell asleep on the back seat. There was no painted center line on the newly paved road. Sudden glaring headlights and screeching brakes confronted them as they rounded a curve in the road. Coming from opposite directions, the two vehicles sideswiped each another.

As the automobiles broadsided, the top of the sleeping Taylor's head apparently smashed into the back left side door post of the car in which he was traveling. He sustained a traumatic injury, creating inordinate swelling and pressure on the upper and lower brain. Driver John Scoble suffered life-threatening bleeding in his lungs, severe injuries to his hip and thigh, and extensive lacerations on his left upper arm and shoulder. Starkly visible scars remain today, thirty-four years later, as John raises his shirt sleeve and recalls the terrifying experience. The individual, riding shotgun, received a comparatively minor cut on his forehead. Subsequently, the three young men were taken by emergency personnel to the Maury County Hospital in Columbia.

When the critical nature of Taylor's and John's injuries was diagnosed at Maury County, the three youths were transported immediately by ambulance to the Trauma Center at Vanderbilt University Medical Center in Nashville, 60 miles north of Columbia. John Scoble, Sr., was the first parent called. It was he who contacted the Colemans in Decatur regarding the accident. Decatur, Alabama, is located 110 miles due south of Nashville, connected by Interstate 65.

An initial 3:45 a.m. evaluation at Vanderbilt was accomplished, and Taylor was taken to surgery for a procedure to relieve the edema pressuring his brain. Within a few hours, a host of other family members and friends, including some of the youth from the conference, began to arrive in the Intensive Care Unit waiting room. A.J. Coleman recalled later having spent that morning with somber visits to the ICU bedside on the one hand and crowd management of distressed visitors on the other.

Through most of Saturday morning, attending physicians were indicating a measured improvement, though Taylor remained gravely ill in a deep coma. As the day wore on, however, Taylor's condition worsened. Though hoping and praying for a positive turnaround, the family was bracing itself for a potentially grim outcome. Shortly after lunch on Saturday, a friend called my home in Nashville to tell me that Taylor, a son of mutual friends A.J. and Shirley Coleman, was in the trauma center at Vanderbilt University Hospital. By the time I arrived in mid-afternoon at the medical center, the more ominous prognosis for Taylor had begun to surface and spirits were at a low point. Late that Saturday evening around midnight, the first of the "flat" EEG (electroencephalograph) tests was clinically noted and reported to the family. Medical indications suggested the possibility of whole-brain death, which included the brain stem.

Those who hover in these somber netherworld gathering places invariably express similar thoughts to one another. Snatched from relatively secure environments, they concur that events are shared there that ordinarily unfold in the lives of other people, not in their own. Initially, their denial bewilders them with hope that they are simply hallucinating or dreaming. Subsequently, they are dragged back to the glaring light of reality by sympathetic medical personnel or spiritual advisors who often must be the bearers of the forbidding and morbid.

As Sunday, July 9, dawned, a weary A.J. and Shirley Coleman and their immediate family were making plans for the day: scheduling respective visits to the ICU bedside, taking incremental periods of rest in nearby accommodations, greeting the many friends and acquaintances who would arrive that day, responding to the plethora of inquiring telephone calls to the waiting room, and having prayers with family and friends. Brian, the Coleman's thirteen-year-old son, was in Nashville with them, and their seven-year-old daughter, Melissa, remained in Decatur with neighbors. En route to lead worship at Donelson Presbyterian Church that Sunday morning, I left home early so that I could briefly visit the Colemans and offer spiritual support and friendship.

Much later on Sunday evening, I shared with my wife, Judy, my uneasiness about retiring for the evening without knowing the status of the young men in the hospital. Earlier that morning the prognosis for Taylor was not good. The likelihood of improvement was slim to nonexistent, so we decided that I should go back to Vanderbilt. Near 10:00 p.m., the usually busy waiting room was almost empty. Mostly, a few family members of other patients in ICU were scattered about, visiting quietly with one another or taking needed catnaps in lounge chairs. Shirley Coleman and her mother, Ethel Braswell, were in their rooms in the Medical Arts Building adjacent to the hospital. Taylor's brother, Brian Coleman, had departed with them. Keeping watch through the night, A.J. and his sister, Sara Pearce, sat together, off to the side in an alcove.

Years later, A.J. reminded me that it wasn't long before Sara and I began an in-depth conversation. That poignant conversation was interrupted at 12:45 a.m. on Monday morning by the even more poignant arrival in the waiting room of the attending physician in neurosurgery at Vanderbilt. His words, contrastingly terse but compassionate, still resonate in my memory after thirty-nine years: "Mr. Coleman, I am so sorry to have to tell you that electroencephalograph indications are that Taylor is brain-dead. You and your family may want to gather once more at his bedside."

With careful elaboration, the physician explained that one "flat" EEG, showing lack of whole-brain function, had been recorded in the chart the night before. Now, a little over twenty-four hours later, another such test registered a similar result. Combined with additional medical indications—pupillary signs, absence of corneal reflexes and ocular movement, absence of gag and cough reflexes, loss of brain-stem function and resultant apnea, it was the confirmation that biological and social death had presented themselves. He could not breathe without the assistance of the respirator. There was no cognitive function or cardio-respiratory capacity. Accordingly, brain-death was determined by the physicians in concert with acceptable medical standards. Withdrawal of the respirator would come next, breathing would cease, and death would be declared.

Since the early 1970s clinical standards included the EEG determinations as well as malfunction of the patient's cardio-respiratory system with the cessation of breathing. Failure of the heart and lungs has been the primary determiner of death for thousands of years, prior to this new technology measuring brain waves. So, significant progress has been made on expanding the criteria for determination of death. However, one could argue, as we will attempt to do in subsequent chapters, that even these criteria for defining death should be expanded to include patients who are clinically determined to be in irreversible *persistent vegetative states*.

The use of the EEG was initiated in the late nineteenth century and further developed in the early twentieth century.[1] It was perfected in the 1930s and was increasingly employed in the 1960s to detect a variety of medical anomalies in the brain such as epilepsy, encephalitis, and anencephaly (babies devoid of upper portions of brain at birth.) Such diagnostic procedures became regularly used, in concert with cardio-respiratory and other medical indications, to determine when a person is dead. Although the EEG was developed for other medical needs, some mentioned above, the critical need for organ transplants became a significant factor in expanded use of the EEG. Blood flow requires the continuation of cardio-pulmonary activity to prevent vegetating organs from imminent damage and deterioration. When spontaneous breathing ceases and the oxygenation of the tissues likewise is terminated, the natural disaster spreads immediately throughout all parts of the body, according to physician Sherwin Nuland: "The stoppage of circulation, the inadequate transport of oxygen to tissues, the flickering out of brain function, the failure of organs, the destruction of vital centers—these are the weapons of every horseman of death."[2] The EEG assists in providing critical information that confirms the diagnosis of severe damage of the brain. No morally driven professional wants to extract organs or tissue from a patient who has the potential for improvement or recovery.

After further conversation with the physician and, mentally and emotionally grasping the situation, A.J. turned to me and asked if I would go to the Medical Arts Building and arouse Brian, Shirley, and Mrs. Braswell. I should escort them back to join other family members for the last plaintive trip to the ICU. Knocking on the door of the young son, mother, and grandmother, I gently whispered the solemn words to Shirley. Then, I waited outside the door while they dressed and with them went to join the other family members. Hand-in-hand we walked together with the chief resident to the holding area adjacent to the ICU.

Taylor was lying on a gurney in an austere anteroom with white linen sheets covering the lower body and feet. Bandages swathed the very top and back of his head. His face and nude upper body bore no sign of injury. A massive bare chest was rising and falling. Shirley Coleman took one look at her son and sobbed hopefully, "Oh, but he's still breathing." A nurse, with tears streaming down her face, stood at the side of the gurney manually operating a portable respirator.

"Yes, he is breathing—artificially," said the physician, "but if the nurse discontinues the manipulation of the respirator, the breathing spontaneously will cease." Then he carefully explained, "Taylor was declared clinically brain-dead in this department. We are assisting the cardio-respiratory function so that the blood supply and oxygen will be delivered to all parts of the body and the kidneys will remain viable, in the hope that you would consent to a transplant. Patients are always waiting in another section of this hospital or another somewhere else to receive such a precious and thoughtful donation of your family in behalf of Taylor, if that is your wish."

With that, A.J. turned to me and emotionally pleaded, "Bob, please help us here; what are your thoughts?" Before I could respond, Taylor's grandmother, Mrs. Braswell, stepped forward.

"Oh, yes," she said softly, "and what about his eyes also?" Years later, A.J. related to me that his main concern was how Mrs. Braswell would deal with donating any of her beloved grandson's body, and that her response immediately put him at ease.

Momentarily, I struggled for words and then said, "The physicians, over the past two days, have been apprising you regularly of the gravity of Taylor's condition. Now, the time of decision has arrived, and we simply have to trust these skilled clinicians that their diagnosis is correct and that already Taylor is in hands that are better than ours, that he is in the hands of God. And what a wonderful gift to consider, parts of his body, to pass on so that other persons can live longer and with a better quality of life."

In the brief space of forty-eight hours, this family learned of a terribly unfortunate accident, experienced a soul-searching hospital vigil, and were confronted with walking away from their respirator-dependent loved one, having acknowledged the destruction of his brain and implicit death. Not only that, they were now faced with a delaying process on removing the respirator and simultaneously granting permission for the donation of Taylor's kidneys and eyes. No one else spoke; there was quiet for a seemingly long thirty to forty seconds until A.J broke the silence: "Then we need to thank God for the gift of Taylor, for the time in which we were privileged to have him as our son and loved one. Let's join hands and pray with God."

A.J. and Shirley Coleman; their youngest son, Brian; A. J.'s sister, Sara Pearce; Taylor's maternal grandmother, Ethel Braswell; the attending physician; and I formed a circle around the gurney. Holding hands with his beloved wife Shirley, this remarkable man of faith led the entire group in prayer, thanking Almighty God for spiritual presence and gifts of life. It was an eternal moment! The only person not holding hands, but who was encircled at the side of Taylor and the gurney, was the tearful nurse manipulating the vital portable respirator.

After the prayer, the gurney was wheeled to a separate transplant unit in a different part of the hospital, where the gift of life was transferred. Paradoxically, the heart was circulating the blood of the brain-dead Taylor, supplying the still-vegetating body parts with its precious oxygen. Although the brain was dead, other parts of the body were not. At the conclusion of a successful transplant, in a separate unit of the hospital, the respirator was removed and breathing ceased along with the flow of blood, which had sustained life, if only incrementally, until that moment. Melissa, Taylor's younger sister, later informed me that his eyes were not transplanted and only one kidney, as the other one was deemed to be too small.

After the transplant of Taylor's organs in the early morning on Monday, July 10, 1972, the condition of the car's driver, John Scoble, stabilized. Later that day, he was transferred from the Critical Intensive Care Unit to a room on the orthopedic floor at Vanderbilt University Medical Center. Because of the life-threatening nature of John's injuries, his family did not initially share with him the fact that his friend Taylor had died. They were no doubt trying to find an appropriate moment for that solemn task, not wanting to add grief to his tenuous medical condition. After John settled into the private room, he asked a family member to secure a radio so that he could listen to music. Ironically, John Scoble heard for the first time on a Nashville news program that his friend Taylor had died with injuries resulting from the tragic accident on a dark road near Columbia, Tennessee. For seven more weeks John remained in his Vanderbilt hospital room, recuperating and contemplating the meaning and purpose of life.

In the 1960s, there were numerous professional groups (medical, legal, philosophical, and theological) that issued studies and statements relative to definitions and determinations of death. As medical technology progressed in that decade with the capacity for delaying the actuality of biological death, the enhanced possibility emerged for organ transplants and related procedures. Thus, it became imperative that medical, moral, and legal directives be forthcoming to prevent legal and moral uncertainty in the clinical setting. A special committee of clinical experts at Harvard Medical School in 1968 called for and produced directives that recognized the total and irreversible loss of whole-brain function as a vital part of declaration of death. It was a significant first step beyond the cardio-respiratory definition in place since the dark ages.

Consequently, the Uniform Determination of Death Act, relative to whole-brain death, was drafted by the National Conference of Commissioners on Uniform State Laws in 1980, in cooperation with the American Medical Association and the President's Commission on Medical Ethics. It was subsequently adopted by religious groups, the American Bar Association, and, ultimately, by all fifty state legislative jurisdictions in the USA. The tragic Taylor Coleman event occurred earlier in 1972, but the essential tenets of those UDDA guidelines were already in place for the physicians and nurses at Vanderbilt bedsides and many other U.S. hospitals.

The brain death of Taylor Coleman was rightly determined by attending neurologists and neurosurgeons in the medical intensive care unit, separately and distinctly from the physicians on the organ recovery team who facilitated the transplant process. In 1973 Catholic Moral Theologian Charles E. Curran wrote appropriately:

> The desire for having organs for transplants runs the risk of breaking the covenant between the doctor and his patient, even though the patient may be dying. The danger exists of declaring a person dead before one would ordinarily do so because of the need of another person for a transplanted organ. Medical ethics, appreciating the pressures on doctors and the weakness of man, calls for a separation of powers between the physician or group who are responsible for the recipient and the physician or group who are responsible for the care of the person who is the prospective donor.[3]

To ensure against professional conflict of interest, interdepartmentally, Vanderbilt's institutional policy and procedure was therefore in concert with the ongoing history of morally relevant transplant protocol. Such policies allay fears of families, or suspicions, that determination of death may be declared too quickly or simply because there are critically ill patients waiting for a potential organ transplant. Taylor Coleman's medical status was thus resolved by his physicians before his transfer to a different department for the removal of organs and the withdrawal of the respirator. The final decision for organ donations was fittingly made by his family. The organ donations were a decision for the family as surrogate to make, in concert with the attending physician. The physicians have the medical and legal right to diagnose and to declare death, but only the patient in advance, or the surrogate, has the right to permit a transplantation procedure. Efforts are currently being made in the United States at medical and legal levels to effect a principle called "presumed consent," allowing for greater numbers of precious organs to be made available for those so desperately awaiting.

Once the actuality of brain death has been clinically established by physicians in the trauma unit, the medically appropriate thing to do is to withdraw all procedures as soon as practicable and to declare that death has occurred. If there are extenuating circumstances, ordinarily I would posit that it is medically, legally, and ethically acceptable to delay shutting off the respirator, even if whole-brain death diagnosis has been declared. In my opinion, "reasonable" delaying procedures should always be negotiable on the part of surrogates and attending physicians. On the other hand, a delay may be requested on the false hope that technology could still rescue the patient or that divine intervention might occur. I would hold that these criteria have no reasonable validity in the clinical setting when the medical indications are conclusive.

Two weeks after the Vanderbilt ICU experience, A.J. and Shirley Coleman returned to Vanderbilt Medical Center Departments of Neurology and Neurosurgery. A case review and discussion ensued with the medical staff, concerning the time line and procedures they earlier shared. One should not be surprised that these parents simply had to know if they and the clinicians had done "the right thing" by walking away from a respirator-dependent Taylor and allowing the transplant surgeons to remove his kidneys and eyes. They were reassured by the medical staff that the appropriate medical and moral choices had been made, given the diagnosis and prognosis presented at that time.

Suffice it to say, deep-seated mental and emotional pangs of what ended and of what might have been still surface in the hearts and minds of A.J. and Shirley Coleman, grim reminders of their netherworld experience. An uncommon anguish is irrevocably impressed upon the heart, mind, and soul of parents when their child of any age precedes them in death. Caregivers, professional and lay, are perpetually challenged by the symptoms of grief that may surface soon or long after any experience of personal loss sustained by individuals.

The National Institute of Neurological Disorders and Stroke estimates that *traumatic* brain injury alone costs the United States more than $56 billion a year. Each year, approximately 1.4 million people experience a TBI, approximately 50,000 people die from head injury, approximately 1 million head-injured people are treated in hospital emergency rooms, approximately 230,000 people are hospitalized for TBI and survive. Additionally, hundreds of American soldiers have died from traumatic brain injuries in the contemporary wars in Iraq and Afghanistan. Thousands more have returned to this country with TBI ranging from mild to very severe, many of which initially are undetected or untreated. The types of tactics and explosives, improvised explosive devices (IEDs) used by terrorists, insurgents, and the Taliban, account for the inordinate rise in these categories because of war-induced injuries to the brain.

Chapter IX

Neocortical Disaster
Persistent Vegetative State

Consistent with the prevailing indicators of death in 1972, medical evaluation of Taylor Coleman's traumatic brain damage was made, donated organs were removed, and supportive technology was withdrawn. Without further delay he was declared dead by whole-brain criteria, irreversible cessation of circulatory/respiratory function, and acceptable medical standards. The standards were clearly delineated and were followed to the letter. Karen Ann Quinlan in 1975, Paul Brophy in 1983, Nancy Cruzan in 1983, and Terri Schiavo in 1990, suffered *non-traumatic* brain injuries, which left them in Persistent Vegetative States (PVS), sustained by medical technology. Though labeled as non-traumatic, the episodes were excessively "hypoxic" in nature, therefore suggesting inadequate or total loss of oxygen flow to the brain for variant periods resulting, in my opinion, in neocortical disaster.[1]

An article in *Medico Legal Neurology* adds strength to the argument: "Many medical conditions result in a brain injury that fails to meet the criteria for brain death, but nevertheless is clearly severe enough to leave the patient permanently incapable of satisfactory recovery."[2] Therefore, languishing in the limbo of medical, legal, moral, and vegetative uncertainty, there is no ready conclusion to the horrible state of existence, that is, no justice for these patients or for their loved ones. "Unfortunately," continues *Medico Legal*, "organ donation is currently impermissible in the absence of full brain death. Despite the logic of expanding the donor pool by including patients in persistent vegetative states, no change on this issue is likely in the near future."[3]

Having earlier seen statistics connected to *traumatic* brain injuries, we cite similar statistics associated with *non-traumatic* brain injuries, provided by the National Institute of Neurological Disorders and Stroke. Credible estimates suggest that, at any given time in the

USA, 10,000–25,000 adults and 6,500–10,000 children lie in a persistent vegetative state with annual costs into the billions.

Compared with the necessarily concise clinical process in the Taylor Coleman case and the expeditiously diagnosed and adjudicated process in the forthcoming Brophy case, I will argue that Quinlan, Cruzan, and Schiavo were, for long periods of time, unjustly left in totally dysfunctional states. Not deemed to be legally dead, they were in my view consigned to states worse than death. It is acknowledged that medical-legal opinions concurred that partially damaged brain cases such as these did not meet definitive criteria for whole-brain death determination. On the other hand, I will contend that the Uniform Definition of Death *itself* did not meet the criteria for bringing *reasonable* certitude and closure for these tragic cases of Quinlan, Brophy, Cruzan, Schiavo, and literally thousands like them.

Beginning with a legal principal, attributable to the nineteenth-century Prime Minister of England William Gladstone, I contend that "justice delayed is justice denied."[4] For more than two decades, argument also has been offered at significant professional levels, that the President's Commission in 1980, and still today, had not gone *far* enough in providing medical, legal, and moral definitions for large numbers of neocortically brain-damaged individuals such as Quinlan, Brophy, and Cruzan.[5] Even with the Uniform Definition of Death in place, clinical settings experience a multiplicity of policies and procedures on responding to episodes of whole or partial brain damage. As if to augment that fact, *Annals of Neurology* in 2007 presented data suggesting that there is a lack of diagnostic uniformity and procedures at the end of life in U.S. hospitals:

> Major differences exist in brain death guidelines among the leading neurological hospitals in the United States. Adherence to the AAN guidelines published in 1995 is quite variable, leading to significant differences in practice which may have consequences for the determination of death and initiation of transplant procedures.[6]

The Terri Schiavo case from 1990 to 2005 dredged up similar concerns and widely diverse professional and lay public debates, provoking significant *individual* and *social* justice issues. My contention is that Schiavo dramatically exerts pressure once more on appropriate professionals in relevant disciplines to consider the need for greater clarity in clinical guidelines on end-of-life issues and specifically for a neocortical definition of death in addition to whole-brain criteria. Philosophers, theologians, and lawyers must bond with medical professionals in applying definitively new brain technologies to the questions of what it means to be a person, to be irreversibly brain damaged, and to be dead.[7] Simultaneously, the necessary triad for the existence of a vigorous national health-care system is one that fosters access, quality, and reasonable cost. Therefore, quality of life at a zero percentile level in thousands of neocortical episodes, impacts the individual and society as a whole, raising a conundrum of medical and fiscal futility in health-care delivery.

In 1994, consecutive special articles entitled, "Medical Aspects of the Persistent Vegetative State." were submitted by The Multi-Society Task Force On PVS, (hereafter, referred to in this manuscript as MSTF).[8] Representing an assortment of neurological societies and associations, this prestigious group of neurological specialists, primarily physicians, accomplished an intensive and thorough examination of what it means to be in a persistent vegetative state. The first of the articles initially explains:

> The term 'persistent vegetative state' was coined by Jeannette and Plum in 1972 to describe the condition of patients with severe brain damage in whom coma has progressed to a state of wakefulness without detectable awareness. Such patients have sleep-wake cycles but no ascertainable cerebral cortical function. Jennette and Plum thought that patients in a persistent vegetative state could be distinguished clinically from those with other conditions associated with prolonged unconsciousness.[9]

At that point in time, though acknowledging the irreversible futility of treating most PVS patients, this MSTF report concluded, "The terms 'neocortical death' and 'apallic state' have limited usefulness and should be abandoned, because they do not represent distinct clinical entities."[10] Much progress in technology and clinical research has occurred over the past decade and a half. Perhaps now, those terms *do* represent "distinct clinical entities." Therefore, I am advocating, along with others, that a professional group similar to the Muti-Society Task Force on PVS serve as a working model for a sorely needed update on this issue of neocortical disaster. Surely the recent and dramatic breakthroughs in brain imaging have taken these issues to a higher and more precise level. Roland Puccetti's argument twenty-seven years ago is considerably more relevant to the present age and is even more promising now in moving beyond a "Whole Brain" definition of death:

> To summarize against Walton on both these points, *for those who have a normal history of neocortical development*, the integrity of the neocortex is essential to the continuance of a mental, and hence a personal life. It follows from this that pallial destruction is equivalent to personal demise, and this has nothing to do with a residual capacity for spontaneous respiration. Thus both the wholly brain dead and the cerebrally dead patient are dead people and it is only superstition to make a vital dichotomy between them.[11]

Though the patient is without sensation or feeling, the extreme or prolonged pain and suffering of the patient's family, however, along with inordinate financial burdens, is a major moral and economic travesty. When continued treatment is futile and offers no medical benefit, allocation of scarce health-care resources is a constant and proliferating distributive justice issue as well.

Quinlan, Brophy, Cruzan, and later Terri Schiavo, sustained devastating non-traumatic upper brain injuries, caused by episodes that led to significant interruption of their vital oxygen supply. Quinlan's lower *brain stem* was only peripherally impacted by the anoxia and later, by court order, she was then removed from a respirator after a brief period of weaning, but remained almost ten years in a persistent vegetative state due to devastation of the neocortex of her brain. Brophy's, Cruzan's and Schiavo's brain stems were unaffected by their respective medical anomalies, but they likewise suffered irreparable damage to the upper brain. All three continued thereupon with beating hearts and no dependence upon respirators. In non-responsive states, however, they were sustained by feeding tubes artificially delivering nutrition and hydration.

Many clinicians, including physicians, philosophers, and theologians, along with this author, raise the question of whether or not a beating heart and vegetating lower body parts alone are enough to confirm meaningful life in persons.[12] Quinlan, Brophy, Cruzan, and Schiavo sustained upper-brain damage that irreparably prevented any return to a cognitive or sapient life. Supported by lower brain (brain stem) activity, their cardio-respiratory systems were functioning, but not one was aware of it.

Both traumatic and non-traumatic brain injuries may result in coma, a state of brief or prolonged unconsciousness. There are diverse extremes in duration and potential outcome when an individual lapses into coma. Depending on the severity of the injury or disease, a person may awaken quickly from the coma, regain consciousness, and return to varying degrees of health. The initial period following an episode is crucial. If the patient does not awaken in several weeks, the likelihood is that she/he will gravitate through an initial vegetative state from which it is still feasible to enter a minimally conscious state and, possibly, a return to consciousness. Contingent upon the cause and severity of an accident or disease, however, most patients with a definitive diagnosis of persistent vegetative state never recover from their cerebral impairment, according to MSTF: "In adults and children with non-traumatic injuries, a persistent vegetative state can be considered to be permanent after three months; recovery does occur, but it is rare and, at best, associated with moderate or severe disability."[13]

One has to assume that neurological specialists have a continuing moral and professional obligation to ferret out and treat those persons who have potential for improvement while being medically realistic about natural limitations and withdrawal of technology from those in diagnosed irreversible comas. Argument is made, on the other hand, that without a definitive medical directive in the form of a more inclusive neocortical definition of death, denial of death proliferates and justice is perpetually denied at individual, social, and distributive levels of health-care delivery. Subsequent cases externalize the argument.

Karen Ann Quinlan

Early in 1975, twenty-one-year-old Karen Ann Quinlan of New Jersey moved out of her parents' home into a house with two friends. It was time for her to demonstrate independence, to seek her livelihood, and, as a young adult, to determine her own destiny. Several months later, after becoming ill and taken by emergency crews to a hospital, in due time Karen was diagnosed by clinicians to be in the morbid medical condition of persistent vegetative state. When initially notified at 2:00 a.m. on April 15, 1975, Julia and Joe Quinlan journeyed forebodingly through the shadowy streets to the Newton Memorial Hospital, where several of their daughter Karen Ann's friends gathered outside the somber emergency department and later in the intensive care waiting room. The more complex Quinlan story was among the first in the United States to initiate ongoing dialogue and litigation on death and dying. This case created a national debate centered upon medical technologies capable of maintaining cerebrally impaired patients for long periods of time on respirators and feeding tubes. Persons would simply have died quickly had not the supportive technology been in place.

Karen Ann's experience started out as a routine evening of celebration among friends at a neighborhood tavern. One of the group was sharing a birthday with the others and, at the outset, the mood was festive. Karen Ann, whom companions reported as being into "starvation" dieting, apparently ingested tranquilizers and small amounts of alcohol on a relatively empty stomach. "And we did find an almost full bottle of Valium in her handbag," reported the intensive care physician, Dr. Paul McGhee. "But that's only a tranquilizer, isn't it?" queried Karen's mother, Julia Quinlan. "It's a tranquilizer," responded the physician. "But the combination of Valium and alcohol are notoriously dangerous."[14] So Karen had become inexplicably lethargic and sleepy. Her friends, perhaps thinking that she was intoxicated, took her to their nearby apartment where she was placed on her bed. A short while later, in checking on her, one of them discovered with alarm that Karen Ann was not breathing. Emergency personnel were called while frantic resuscitation efforts, with minimal results, were made to revive her.

No one really knows for certain how long Karen Ann was without cardio-pulmonary circulation. A later court record says that she "ceased breathing for at least two 15 minute periods."[15] What is known, for certain, is that four-and-a-half minutes or more without life-sustaining oxygen flowing through the body to the brain and other tissues, is a formula for destruction. With anoxic deprivation, the critically important centers are quickly impacted and the oxygen-divested brain suffers irreversible deterioration. The combination of tranquilizer, several cocktails, and scant food in Karen Ann's stomach from dieting, was apparently a lethal mixture which, in her case, contributed to cardiac arrest.

Subsequently, at Newton Memorial Hospital, Karen Ann Quinlan, in 1975, was diagnosed with "irreversible brain damage." Nine days later, still unconscious and on a respirator, she was transferred to St. Clare's Hospital in Denville, New Jersey. Constant bedside vigils were maintained by Karen's parents, Joe and Julia Quinlan, her two siblings Mary Ellen and John, and a host of friends. The devout Roman Catholic family, initially facing their ordeal, was nurtured by the presence of their faithful parish priest, The Rev. Father Tom Trapasso, as well as other spiritual counselors through the years.

Karen Ann's parents were reluctant to accept the ominous medical diagnosis and initially believed that her condition might improve. However, the later prognosis of PVS raised vital questions of maintaining life by machines, a prospect that the parents knew fervently in their hearts that Karen Ann would not have wanted. Earlier family discussions, in fact, had been held precisely on that issue. Then, Father Trapasso's interpretation of the Catholic Bishop's Health Care Directives affirmed that the church law did not force the use of extraordinary respirator support to prolong natural life.[16] After several months of emotional and spiritual struggle, on July 31, 1975, the family requested that St. Clare physician, Robert Joseph Morse, M.D. and hospital staff withdraw the respirator: "Knowing Karen we all realize that she would never want to be kept alive in this way. She would agree with what we are deciding tonight." After the meeting with the family, "Dr. Morse stood up then, and he put his hand on Joe's shoulder and said sympathetically, 'I think you've made the right decision.' "[17]

Though the attendant physician initially agreed to honor the written request signed by Karen's father, overnight he changed his mind. Near mid-morning the next day he called Joe Quinlan at his office and said, "Joe, I have a moral problem about what we agreed on last night. I feel that I have to consult someone else and see how *he* feels about it."[18] At the next meeting of the family with the physician and administrative staff, a lawyer representing the physician's and hospital's legal interests was present.

In fairness to the physicians and hospital involved, it is true that the lines that established medical morality and legality were dramatically blurred at this point in U.S. history. Science had impacted clinical settings, allowing procedures that theretofore were not possible and that were neither sufficiently adjudicated nor morally evaluated at the time. The Nazi regime, the Holocaust, and their accompanying medical atrocities, I would argue, had influenced not only medical research but clinical bedside procedures in the United States and around the world.[19]

For the physician and hospital administration to have second thoughts about withdrawing support systems, in my view, was not unusual given the uncertainty of the period concerning end-of-life issues. Physician paternalism was prevalent at that time, while clinical procedures allowing patient and surrogate choice were in their larval stages. With every new technology complex issues were surfacing and raising new questions. Some clinicians debated that there were cases, such as this one, in which it was better to err on the side of caution or safety (tutioristic view). Even the United Sates Supreme Court initially suggested caution when ruling on the Cruzan case, which follows this one, upholding Missouri's "clear and convincing evidence standard."[20] Without a doubt, careful scrutiny and patience at the bedside are indeed attitudes of first choice—but scrutiny and patience may also lead to other decisions based on solid medical and moral evidence that withholding and withdrawing care are appropriate procedures and are consistent with the predetermined wishes of the patient or surrogate.

The physician in the Quinlan case, from legal and moral perspectives, no doubt was concerned about criminal complicity and about what constitutes euthanasia. He was supported in that view by the current clinical standards existing at that point in New Jersey. Since Karen did not show flat EEG brain waves and was displaying vegetative responses, she did not meet the Harvard University criteria for whole-brain death, accepted at that point in many legal jurisdictions. Though applicable for the Taylor Coleman case, I have submitted at the same time that it was self-evident that the Harvard definition for death and the later Uniform Definition of the Presidential Commission were inadequate themselves when applied to the cases like the one of Karen Ann Quinlan, and thus it becomes a justice issue.

My opinion is that the Quinlans were justified in their frustration with the reneging of the physicians, along with the policies and procedures of the St. Clare Hospital, the Harvard University criteria for whole-brain death, and the laws of the state of New Jersey. This family believed that none of those entities were serving fairly Karen Ann's best interest, and I am in moral and legal support of that belief. By the time of the next meeting with hospital staff, the Quinlans had acquired a bright young lawyer to represent Karen Ann and themselves, Paul W. Armstrong, Esquire, Attorney for the Plaintiff. Joe Quinlan had gone to the Dover, New Jersey Legal Aid Society to acquire guardianship for Karen. That visit led several days later to the attorney for that agency resigning his job to represent Karen and the Quinlans in their legal effort to have Karen's respirator removed.[21] His telephone call to Joe Quinlan indicated that he would accept the case pro bono (without fee). The young attorney, along with his wife, recognized the legal magnitude of this case and the professional recognition and ultimate benefits he would receive in arguing the case before the New Jersey Supreme Court.

Joe Quinlan and his lawyer subsequently went into a New Jersey Superior Court for relief in behalf of his daughter. He wanted remediation for his daughter, which she could not seek for herself from within her brain-damaged state. Actually, she had shared thoughts with her family about situations like the one eventually impacting her own life. Later courts accepted such expressions as ones of self-determination. They were considered unwritten advance directives, statements of values applicable to the principle of autonomy. This case was, however, a unique one as suggested at that time by ethicist Robert Veatch:

> In most situations of the sort, there is quiet agreement between parents and guardians and physicians usually with doctors making suggestions that the family accepts. What is unusual here is that the parents are taking the initiative, and that is how it should be. In

my opinion the parents, as next of kin, ought to have the option to make such a tough choice. Since Karen does not have 'brain death,' the case moves into a gray area of ethics and law, where no precedent exits.[22]

Joe Quinlan's petition to a New Jersey Superior Court was denied, however, by Judge Robert Muir on the basis that Karen Ann's condition did not meet the Harvard criteria for brain death and current medical standards on withholding and withdrawing issues. He also ruled that Karen was a twenty-one-year-old adult, and the state had guardianship rights, not the plaintiff, Joe Quinlan.

It is clear to me that this family believed that none of those entities were serving fairly Karen Ann's best interest. My argument is that the medical and legal systems were failing them in not providing timely relief for Karen Ann's plight, and apparently her family thought so as well. Karen and her family needed forthright relief from the respirator, which they believed offered no immediate or future benefit for her in her then present state. Thus, the ruling was appealed to the New Jersey Supreme Court by Joe Quinlan and his lawyer on a different point of law, the perceived basis of Karen Ann's constitutional right to privacy. This effectively bypassed the state attorney general's concern that, under then current statutes, respirator removal from a patient not "whole-brain" dead, might constitute criminal homicide. The state Supreme Court also found correctively, I would concur, that the lower court erred in its award of Karen Ann's guardian rights to the state as opposed to her family, which was in a better position to act in her best interest.[23]

The U.S. Constitution clauses respecting privacy, therefore, nudged the New Jersey Supreme Court to overturn the lower court to grant the permission of respirator removal. But, the ruling was based on the condition that the St Clare Hospital "ethics committee" and the attendant physicians concur on the irreversibility of her vegetative state, that is, the improbability of a return to a cognitive, sapient state. In any event, the respirator was removed. The ethics guideline established by the New Jersey Supreme Court in the Quinlan case thus resulted in an almost immediate increase in the placement of, and later a requirement for, ethics advisory committees in most clinical settings throughout the United States. At the same time, the New Jersey Supreme Court decision in Quinlan was a catalyst for spreading interest in and concern for advance directives, which give support for a patient's right to autonomy. Somewhat later, the Joint Commission, which monitors and grants accreditation to most U.S. hospitals, offered a guideline in its directives that required a mechanism for dealing with such ethical issues, including, but not limited to, ethics advisory committees.

With apparent minimal damage to her brain stem and subsequent surprise to her family, Karen Ann did not stop breathing when the respirator was withdrawn. Even though neocortically devastated, having sustained irreversible damage to both cerebral hemispheres with permanently lost cognition, Karen Ann's intact brain stem kept her cardio-respiratory system functional for almost nine more years! At another time and in another place, the longest such "vegetative case" ever recorded, lasted for 37 years and 111 days.[24] One year after the initial insults to *her* brain, Karen Ann was described in the appeals court record as "emaciated, having suffered a weight loss of at least 40 pounds, and undergoing a continuing deteriorative process. Her posture is described as fetal-like and grotesque; there is extreme flexion, rigidity of the arms, legs, and related muscles, and her joints are severely rigid and deformed."[25]

Karen Ann existed in a vegetative state with no socio-relational capacity. She received nutrition and hydration artificially through a plastic tube and experienced sleep-wake cycles—at times with eyes closed in an apparent peaceful state—at other times intermittently opening her eyes but never focusing, while grimacing, groaning, and gnashing! Physician Daniel Dilling comments on the broad misinterpretation of this medical phenomenon:

> A clearer understanding of the diagnostic criteria for PVS is needed, for both the medical community and the lay public, as we ponder this issue. The open eyes and presence of autonomic function can be both confusing and bothersome for the families and healthcare personnel and can lead to false expectations and flawed decisions.[26]

Though sleep/wake/intermittently open eyes wrongly suggested otherwise, Karen Ann had no cerebral awareness of her family's presence, nor did she ever know pain, hunger, thirst, fear, anxiety, or loneliness. Mentally and spiritually she was in another sphere of existence, although enabled by technology to remain vegetatively in this one. In the midst of the legal and religious posturing on what constituted juridical precedence and church practice, the medical issue was the improbability of Karen Ann's return to a cognitive and sapient state.

Clinical realties indicated that there was no reasonable medical benefit to be derived from maintenance of the artificial nutritional and hydrational support systems. The MSTF of physicians and ethicists states:

> When artificial nutrition and hydration are withdrawn, patients in a persistent vegetative state usually die within 10 to 14 days. The immediate cause of death is dehydration and electrolyte imbalance rather than malnutrition; patients in a persistent vegetative state cannot experience thirst or hunger.[27]

The Quinlan family and their religious directives, however, considered nutritional and hydrational support to be *ordinary* necessities that should be maintained as long as Karen Ann was breathing. The Roman Catholic Church ethical and religious directives defines the respirator as *extraordinary* treatment, which could be withheld or withdrawn, but places nutrition and hydration at a more basic need level, one which should be maintained, even though the patient exists in a brain-damaged state with no capacity for hunger or thirst. That church body's teaching on the extraordinary distinction flows from a 1957 pronouncement by Pope Pious II, which remains intact under the authorization of the current Pope Benedict XVI. I would argue that there should be no medical, moral, or legal distinction separating the respirator and the feeding tube, a view that is held also by some contemporary Catholic theologians. One such ethicist is Daniel Maguire. Professor of Moral Theology at Marquette University, a Catholic Jesuit institution:

> The respirator is, of course, an extraordinary means especially when it is used on the irreversibly unconscious. For years now theologians have also argued that even intravenous feeding in this type of

case is extraordinary and may be discontinued.... To maintain bodily life extensively at a vegetative level with extraordinary means is irrational, immoral, and a violation of the dignity of human life.[28]

Two months into her tenth year of vegetative state, Karen Ann once again developed pneumonia, the most common cause of death with persons in PVS. On June 11, 1985, Karen Ann Quinlan succumbed to the pneumonia and respiratory failure. So to remove only the respirator did not solve the problem. It created for Paul and Julia Quinlan the moral dilemma of having to choose between what they believed were two equally undesirable courses of action. They could leave brain-damaged Karen Ann in a vegetative state, which decision they ultimately chose. Or they could have decided on the alternative, withdrawing the nutrition and hydration and allowing a natural death. To have chosen the latter, they believed, would have violated Roman Catholic moral law. I cannot fault them for remaining faithful to the teachings of their church. I can only express regrets that there is such ethical dissonance separating their faith tradition from those who believe that there is no moral distinction separating the technology of respirators and feeding tubes.

Neocortical Death

Philosophy Professor John Lachs of Vanderbilt University stated twenty-five years ago:

> When we unalterably lose the ability to will and to do, to think and to hope, to feel and love, we have ceased existence as human beings. The only humane course then is to declare us dead and to treat us accordingly. If the diagnosis is careful and accurate, we need have no fear that this harms anyone: once the human person is gone, in the faltering body there is no one there.[29]

Shortly after becoming appointed to the adjunct faculty with Professor Richard M. Zaner at Vanderbilt University Medical Center and its Center for Clinical and Research Ethics, I was involved there in an ethics symposium on October 18-20, 1984. Respected physicians, nurses, lawyers, philosophers, and other medical ethicists offered formal presentations and led discussions on the topic: "When Are You Dead?: Critical Appraisals of Whole-Brain and Neocortical Definitions of Death." Dr. Lachs' observations were part of his presentation at the symposium and were later published in 1988 with other theses in the significant book *Death: Beyond Whole-Brain Criteria,* edited by Dr. Zaner.[30] At that time, Zaner was Stahlman Professor of Medical Ethics at Vanderbilt University School of Medicine and Director of the Center for Clinical and Research Ethics. Also participating was Attorney-Ethicist Alexander Capron, the Executive Director of the President's Commission, which drafted the original Whole-brain Determination of Death statement.[31]

In the Vanderbilt symposium, conceived and facilitated by Dr. Zaner, a majority of the presenters, along with Zaner himself, essentially concluded that the President's Commission was deficient in its recommended Uniform Determination of Death Act (UDDA). The presidential task force, they said, simply did not go far enough in its mission to answer succinctly the question, "When is a person dead?" In calling for the symposium, Zaner took to task the President's Commission by arguing, "The kind of patient which the commission and other 'whole brain' advocates took as the paradigm for defining death, however, is distinctly different from those in a 'persistent vegetative state.'"[32] Most presenters at the forum agreed that there should be other definitive statements that include a sorely needed standard for acknowledging "neocortical death" as well. Much has been discussed and written since then on this very complex subject. For those interested in a classic discussion on the issues involved, however, a starting place might very well be the book edited by Richard Zaner.

In addition to John Lachs and significant others in the 1984 Vanderbilt Symposium, and contributors to the Zaner-edited book, were Edward T. Bartlett, Ph.D., and Stuart Youngner, M.D., who concluded, "Death is not the loss of something to someone; it is the loss of some one. Because a human being is a person, the irreversible destruction of the neocortex—i.e., the center of consciousness and cognition, constitutes death."[33] These were the functions, irretrievably lost in the brain of Karen Ann Quinlan and later in the brains of

Howard Brophy, Nancy Cruzan, and Terri Schiavo. Philosopher Robert Veatch, essentially in concert with Bartlett and Youngner, states, "I shall defend in this paper a higher brain concept. By that I mean that a person should be considered dead when there is an irreversible loss of higher brain functions—i.e., certain functions normally associated with the neocortex that include the capacity to be conscious, to think, to feel, and to be aware of other people."[34]

As part of his rationale for chiding the President's Commission on its inadequate determination of death statement, philosopher Robert Veatch said, "For a country that stands so close to the Judeo-Christian tradition, to reject the position favored by that tradition and by most contemporary scholars within that tradition seems odd."[35] Veatch's reference here is to the Biblical concept of the "conjoining of body and soul—or to use the more modern language, mind and body." Thus, I would agree substantially with him on his view of the importance of "unity of mind and body."[36]

The Council of Theology and Culture of the Presbyterian Church U.S. in 1981, (before its merger with the Presbyterian Church, (U.S.A.) in 1983) presented a concept of such "interrelatedness" for adoption at its General Assembly. In responding to an injunction by its highest court that it reflect on the nature and value of human life, the council issued a statement with which I concur:

> Human life is distinguished in the biblical narrative by it relations of mutuality to God and to other human beings. Without these relationships the reality we know as human life does not come into the Bible's focus. . . . Thus mutual relatedness belongs not only to the well-being of human life, but to its very being.[37]

So much, therefore, depends on one's definition of death and the use, by Professor Lachs, of the word *if*—"*If* the diagnosis is careful and accurate," he said, "we need have no fear that this harms anyone."[38] Such fear and at times panic, however, were a significant part of the historical perspective delivered by Dr. Martin S. Pernick of the University of Michigan in his opening remarks at the 1984 symposium at Vanderbilt and their place in the first chapter of the book edited by Zaner. The title of Pernick's fascinating presentation was revealing: "Back from the Grave: Recurring Controversies over Defining Death and Diagnosing Death in History." Two observations and a final enjoinder by Dr. Pernick stand out among much historical data worthy of note: "Death has never been completely definable in objective technical terms. It has always been at least in part a subjective and value-based construct."[39] Thus, from the very beginning of Western history, defining and diagnosing death proved both perplexing and controversial."[40]

We applaud Dr. Pernick's thorough review of the historical data which point to the complexities of defining and diagnosing death through the centuries, complexities resurging in the twenty-first century as new technologies create new ethical dilemmas and more complex uncertainties. To suggest that these issues have been and are, both "perplexing and controversial," should not surprise anyone, given the social and political turmoil erupting over the recently controversial and sad Terri Schiavo case. But, relative to the potential adoption of a definition of neocortical death, Dr. Pernik offers a concluding proviso in the book, the publication of which followed the Vanderbilt forum. "By analogy with such precedents, if 'higher brain' definitions are not currently capable of being rigorously operationalized, it may be socially harmful and therefore premature to promote them."[41]

There may be some truth in that, but there have been twenty-eight years now since the whole brain definition was placed before the nation, and annually there have been thousands of neocortically damaged patients in that period of time, loved ones whose families have desperately sought medical and legal closure similar to that offered by the whole-brain definition of death. In the face of pleas for medical and moral justice, I continually argue along with the others mentioned that it is reasonable and timely for appropriate professionals to present a "higher brain" standard for the determination of death in irreparably brain-damaged patients. As many competent authorities have recommended, we must move beyond whole-brain criteria to proliferate the transfer to others of vital body parts through transplantation—and subsequently, removal of life support systems to allow the natural death of these persons. Without such a higher brain standard, justice is being delayed and, in my opinion, a culture of death denial will remain constant or will proliferate, as the forthcoming case of Terri Schiavo in this manuscript suggests.

Also, another related issue mentioned by Dr. Pernick troubled me throughout the symposium at Vanderbilt and ever since. There are some who believe, he said in his lecture, "To kill one patient is worse than continued treatment of 1000 corpses." Though not personally endorsing the statement, Dr. Pernick did refer to the view within the context of the historical data that set the stage for later forum discussion. He also stated that in the closing decades of the nineteenth century there was a panic that one's own self might be the victim of premature burial. I would submit that there seems to have been, in the opening decade of the twenty-first century, a panic that withholding or withdrawing technology might lead to the premature declaration of death of oneself or some other or person.

My fear is not that I or others, hovering in a persistent vegetative state, will be diagnosed with irreversible brain damage and therefore consigned to a premature burial or cremation because of an expansive definition of death. Contrarily, my concern is that mine and thousands of other "breathing corpses"[42] might languish technologically in clinical settings throughout this land because of a sharply limited definition of death. If that were to happen, my family and others would be subjected to chronic despair and long-term financial deprivation. Therefore, I steadfastly argue for withdrawing treatment and acknowledging the immanence of natural death in cases of clearly diagnosed cases of persistent vegetative state. This is a major premise throughout this book based on autonomy, the right of the individual to medical self-determination, and, subsequently, the right to justice for oneself and for one's neighbor.

Many would contend forcefully that we have a right to life. I would respond just as vociferously, along with Sherwin Nuland, that we also have a reasonable right to our own death[43]—that we as a society are obligated to give persons, in the face of medically exacerbating and futile situations, the privilege of refusing treatment, allowing them to die. As long as such persons are deemed mentally competent, such an autonomous request may be implemented through personal demonstration or in advance through written directives. Brain damaged or mentally incompetent patients may receive equally just treatment through an appropriately determined surrogate acting in accordance with their wishes or in their best interest. This right to personal autonomy in medical issues, as noted earlier, was enacted by congress in 1990, the Patient Self-Determination Act, becoming effective in 1991.

As we have seen, brain injury can emanate from both *traumatic* and *non-traumatic* causes. At that level, there has been logical caution among clinicians in asserting that a patient has arrived at a diagnosis of irreversible neocortical destruction and persistent vegetative state. Ordinarily, many weeks or months (sometimes years) of clinical observation and treatment are involved before such a declaration. Furthermore, added to the diagnostic formulae are new imaging scan techniques such as Positron Emission Tomography (PET), Computed Tomography (CT), and Functional Magnetic Resonance Imaging (FMRI). In 1992 Professor Robert Rakestraw argued,

> Although PET scans are done in relatively few centers across America and are moderately costly, a much more widely available and less costly procedure the pulsed Doppler ultrasound (PDU) test may be utilized. . . . The PDU measurement of the carotid artery blood flow is accurate by itself and can be done in any hospital in America. Schernmer calls this a 'landmark discovery: the actual clinical point of death of the human being can now be identified technologically with certainty. If there is still some question, PET studies of cerebral blood flow and glucose metabolism give further confirmation of whether or not the patient's cortex is definitely dead.[44]

These medical marvels are literally opening the deep secrets of the brain and have uncovered problematic conditions that, heretofore, were medically untreatable—thus the ongoing potential for dramatic continuation of treatment and possible cures on the one hand, while on the other, allaying the fears that withholding or withdrawing treatment might be prematurely determined. These advanced technologies have the capability to assess cerebral damage and deterioration; none thus far has the capacity for reversal or cure for PVS. Irreparable upper brain malfunction, combined with other medical indications and imaging procedures, including total incapacity for responding to mental and physical stimulation, ordinarily leaves no doubt in the minds of neurological experts when accidents or disease have irreparably accomplished their destructive mission. Professor/Attorney/Ethicist David Smith thus contends:

> Arguably, the right-to-die cases involving irreversibly unconscious patients already establish a medical and legal precedent because expert physicians repeatedly have testified with confidence that the patients involved in the particular cases were irreversibly unconscious and insentient.[45]

> As greater numbers of neocortically dead patients undergo PET scans, medical scientists will be able to formulate levels of bio-energetic chemical utilization below which persons do not ever regain consciousness. In short, with the break-through in PET scanning, it is no longer tenable to argue that neocortical death is incapable of being reliably diagnosed.[46]

That it is medically, philosophically, legally, ethically, and theologically appropriate to withhold and to withdraw non-beneficial treatment from persons in such profoundly questionable cases continues to be my steadfast conclusion and that of many clinical ethicists in the mainstream of clinical ethics. On the issue of neocortical disaster we appear to be in accord with Zaner, Spicker, Veatch, Puccetti, Engelhardt, Smith, Bartlett, Youngner, and many others who are prepared to say with Lachs, "The only humane course is to declare us dead and to treat us accordingly."[47]

Professor Lachs's assertion that persons in irreversibly flawed brain states should be declared dead is decidedly a humane one. But I would suggest an adjunctive course that is even more humane, that is, assertively sharing the still viable body parts before making the declaration and withdrawing the support systems. I am certain that he would agree. Organs, eyes, bone, and tissue, the residue of fatally flawed body systems, are desperately needed by thousands of persons who would greatly benefit through vastly expanded transplantation efforts. Thus, Mary Moore's Vanderbilt Medical Center bed sign takes on greater relevance, "Don't Bury Organs—Recycle Them."[48]

Chapter X

PVS

(Continuation)

Nancy Beth Cruzan

On a cold, January 11, 1983, day in Jasper County near Carthage, Missouri, an automobile traveling on a narrow, curving, slick road flipped upside down into a ditch near a grove of trees. Someone living nearby heard the crash, investigated, and called state troopers and medical emergency personnel, who arrived rather quickly. The driver of the wrecked car was a twenty-five-year-old woman named Nancy Beth Cruzan, whom the paramedics found to be unconscious, in cardiac arrest, and therefore not breathing. Subsequently, they were able to resuscitate her. At the hospital she remained unresponsive but, with lower brain stem activity, was able to breathe on her own. As with Quinlan though, it was necessary to insert a feeding tube into her stomach for artificial nutrition and hydration in order for her to survive.

Court documents provide estimates from witnesses and emergency personnel that indicated that Nancy had been without cardio-respiratory activity for a period of time, twelve to fourteen minutes. The Missouri trial court in this case found that permanent brain damage generally results after six minutes in an anoxic state.[1] She was deprived of oxygen until resuscitated at the roadside and taken to a local hospital. Several months later, the young woman was diagnosed with irreversible neocortical brain damage, as non-sentient and in a persistent vegetative state. She lay in fetal position, exhibited typical sleep/wake cycles, facial grimaces, bodily contortions, and issued guttural sounds. Like Karen Ann Quinlan, there was absolutely no awareness or other cerebral activity. Nancy was maintained in the vegetative condition until, by court order, her feeding tube was removed almost eight years later on December 14, 1990—but not until legal process had taken place in the Jasper County Missouri Circuit Court, the Missouri Supreme Court, the United States

Supreme Court, and back again to the court of original jurisdiction, the Jasper County Circuit Court (probate division) of Judge Charles E. Teel, Jr.

In the meantime, between January 1983 and December 1990, court documents show that twenty-five-year-old Nancy was placed in a Missouri State Rehab Hospital by her parents of modest means.[2] Though granted legal guardianship, they were not deemed responsible for the hospital expenses, which were estimated at $130,000 annually over an almost eight-year period. Since she was past the age of twenty-one and disabled, like Quinlan in New Jersey, she was made a legal ward of the state of Missouri, which assumed the million-dollar total cost of her care under its federally mandated Medicaid Program. As a ward of the state, therefore, a guardian ad litem was appointed by the court to serve in the best interest of the hapless individual, even though her family was in a constantly supportive role.

After demonstrating five and a half years of faithfulness at the bedside of their daughter, Lester and Joyce Cruzan finally sought medical and legal relief for Nancy and themselves. In July of 1988, Jasper County Circuit Court Judge Charles E. Teel, Jr., ruled that previous conversations with family and friends were "clear and convincing evidence" that Nancy would not have wanted to remain in such a vegetative state, with irreversible brain damage and permanent loss of cognition. The nutrition and hydration support could be removed.[3]

So, at least temporarily, the law came to the medical, legal, and moral rescue of Nancy Cruzan and her family. She was fettered by technology and lay in a non-sentient vegetative state. Judge Teel legally affirmed Nancy's right to privacy—the right to be left alone—the right, through her surrogate, to refusal or withdrawal of treatment. Though in a brain-damaged state, Nancy's claim to autonomy, as with Karen Ann Quinlan, was made in advance through conversation with her family and was recognized and, in my opinion, was fairly adjudicated by Judge Teel. The perceptions of George Annas, commenting retrospectively after the legal struggle preceding the death of Terrie Schiavo in 2005, are pertinent to the earlier Cruzan case in 1988:

The law has been remarkably stable since *Quinlan* (which itself restated existing law): competent adults have the right to refuse any medical treatment, including life-sustaining treatment (which includes artificially delivered fluids and nutrition). Incompetent adults retain an interest in self-determination. Competent adults can execute an advance directive stating their wishes and designate a person to act on their behalf, and physicians can honor these wishes. Physicians and health-care agents should make treatment decisions consistent with what they believe the patient would want (subjective standard). If the patient desires cannot be ascertained, then treatment should be based on the patient's best interests (what a reasonable person would most likely want in the same circumstances). This has, I believe, always been the law in the United States.[4]

The Cruzan's lower court victory proved to be short-lived, however, and I would argue that the law proved to be inadequate for Nancy Cruzan at this time as it had been for Karen Ann Quinlan for over a decade. Again, it was a case of justice denied, due to the delay of justice. "Although *Quinlan* was widely followed," observed Annas later in 2005, "the New Jersey Supreme Court could make law only for New Jersey."[5] With strong legal commitment to sanctity of life over quality of life, therefore, the guardian ad litem, acting in the absence of the Missouri State Attorney General, appealed Judge Teel's ruling to the State Supreme Court. That court acknowledged that Nancy Beth Cruzan's "brain has degenerated" and that her "cerebral cortical atrophy is irreversible, progressive, and ongoing." Even so, by a vote of four to three, the higher Missouri court, in November of 1988, reversed the lower court's decision, preventing the removal of medical treatment in the form of nutrition and hydration tubes. In dissenting, Judge Welliver viewed the conversations of Nancy and her family as tantamount to presenting advance directives and declared:

> If we cannot authorize withdrawing or withholding 'medication,' 'nutrition,' or 'hydration,' then what can

we authorize to be withheld in Missouri? The Missouri Living Will Act is a fraud on Missourians who believe we have been given a right to execute a living will, and to die naturally, respectably, and in peace.[6]

The submitted evidence, as related to Nancy's earlier conversations with her family were considered not "compelling" enough to meet Missouri's more stringent interpretation of "clear and convincing" evidence. The Missouri legislature earlier had passed legislation permitting the removal of some life support systems. However, they did not approve of withholding and withdrawing nutrition and hydration sustenance in clinical settings and the Supreme Court's split its decision. I argue, therefore, that it unfairly subordinated Nancy Cruzan's values and right to medical autonomy as stated by her to friends and family months before her tragic accident. Courts, like any other human institution, can err, and it is the responsibility of other courts, along with philosophers and theologians, to take them to task when they do.

William Colby, attorney for the Cruzans, urged them to take the case to the Supreme Court of the United States, believing their appeal to have merit and that the timing was right. His argument, no doubt, was that the widespread debates on death with dignity, along with concurring natural death legislation in Missouri and other state jurisdictions, might open the door for the nation's highest court to consider their case. He was correct. Cruzan became the first "right to die" case to be heard on appeal to the U.S. Supreme Court. But the decision, handed down on June 23, 1990, *initially* was a setback for Attorney Colby and favored the state of Missouri over the Cruzans, on the basis of its "clear and convincing evidence requirement." Nancy remained in a persistent vegetative state, being sustained artificially through a tube placed in her stomach.

The ruling by the U.S. Supreme Court affirmed that it is the patient's unilateral decision, not anyone else's, to have treatment withheld or withdrawn—not that of the family, the physician, or the state! That is consistent with the overriding principle of autonomy, applicable here to Nancy's previous conversations with her family. However, the lower court evidence of what Nancy might have wanted was deemed earlier by Missouri's highest court to be insufficient, short of written statements, despite the testimony of family and friends. The U.S. Supreme Court upheld Missouri in its "clear and convincing evidence" requirement but, at the same time, found strong support for the use of living wills and other advance directives, which, I would argue also, intensifies the importance of this case and enhances the value of the conversations that Nancy experienced with family and friends.

Simultaneously, the U.S. Supreme Court did more! Justice Sandra O'Conner joined the majority of the court in affirming that nutrition and hydration tubes are, in fact, medical treatments that can legally be withheld or withdrawn. In her concurrence she states, "artificial feeding cannot readily be distinguished from other forms of medical treatment."[7] That opinion foreshadowed a turnabout for the Cruzan's legal interface with the state of Missouri.

Following the June 1990 court decision in Washington, Lester and Joyce Cruzan returned to Jasper County with their attorney, William Colby. Once more, with additional witnesses, they filed briefs in Judge Teel's circuit court requesting that Nancy's feeding tube be removed. This time the state withdrew from the case and did not appeal Judge Teel's decision that all medical treatment, including the artificial feeding tube, be terminated—a ruling based on "clear and convincing" evidence of what Nancy Cruzan would have wanted. Judge Teel got it right for the second time, and George Annas was able to observe retrospectively, "When the U.S. Supreme Court decided the case of Nancy Cruzan, in 1990, it made constitutional law for the entire country."[8] Justice was finally served, and Judge Teel was vindicated in his earlier verdict, an acknowledgement of Nancy's earlier conversations with family as being "clear and convincing evidence" of what she would have wanted, if involved in same or similar circumstances.

The Cruzan case accomplished for **feeding tubes** what Quinlan had done for **respirators**. Both artificial supports are now considered by the courts to be medical interventions which may be withheld or withdrawn when they no longer provide a reasonable medical benefit, particularly when the withholding and withdrawal conforms to the predetermined wishes of the patient. Nancy Cruzan's accident resulted in a brain-damaged persistent vegetative state. Her previous conversations with family members enabled her surrogate to testify in her behalf as to what her wishes might be if, subsequently, she might be found in such a state.

Therefore, in a journal article appearing in May 1991, Dr. Bruce D. White, et al, appropriately substantiated the importance of patient autonomy, written advance directives, conversations with family, and the appointment of surrogates, when the patients lose sentience and can no longer speak for themselves: "Essentially, the *Cruzan* decision provides federal constitutional validation to three decades of work in medicine and medical ethics that has shifted the paradigm from a traditional paternalistic one to an increasing emphasis on patient prerogatives to make their own health-care decisions."[9]

Nancy Cruzan had remained in a persistent vegetative state for almost eight years. She was declared dead on December 26, 1990, twelve days after the artificial feeding tube was removed from her stomach. Before and after the removal of the tube, Nancy experienced no awareness of hunger, thirst, discomfort, pain, or loneliness, due to the neocortical damage to her brain. She was thirty-two years of age. On her cemetery tombstone are engraved words that speak of the dire cerebral episode occurring seven years earlier on January 11, 1983. The event ultimately consigned her to the physical and mental imprisonment of the persistent vegetative and with it the loss of her sentient being:[10]

Nancy Beth Cruzan
**Most Loved
Daughter—Sister—Aunt
Born July 20, 1957
Departed January 11, 1983
At Peace December 26, 1990**

Other closely related patient rights events took place in Washington concurrently with the Cruzan legal struggles. Episcopal priest John Danforth, the Republican Senator from Missouri (1976-1994), had followed the unjust plights of Karen Ann Quinlan in New Jersey, his Missouri constituent Nancy Cruzan, and thousands of others nationwide. Thus, he crafted legislation, named it the Patient Self-Determination Act, and steered it through the U.S. Congress as part of the Omnibus Budget Reconciliation Act of 1990.

The federal law, which became effective on December 1, 1991, was essentially directed toward health-care providers and suppliers. They are required to provide patients with information relative to six specific issues, the most important of which are twofold: (1) the patient's right to accept or refuse medical or surgical procedures; (2) documentation in the patient's medical record as to whether or not the individual executed an advance directive on accepting, refusing, or withdrawing medical treatment (Living Will and/or Durable Power of Attorney for Health Care).

Prior to the important Quinlan (1976) and Cruzan (1990) cases, a number of legal cases through the years had already fed a growing support in the law for medical self-determination and the right to die. Three of those, among many others, are Union Pacific Company vs. Botsford 1891, Mohr vs. Williams in 1905, and Schloendorff vs. Society of New York Hospitals in 1914. The U.S. Supreme Court, on Botsford, agreed in the majority with Justice Gray: "No right is held more sacred, or is more carefully guarded by the common law, than the right of every individual to the possession and control of his own person, free from all restraint or interference of others, unless by clear and unquestionable authority of law."[11] In the Mohr case the ruling read in part, "The free citizen's first and greatest right, which underlies all others, is the right to himself."[12] Then, in Schloendorff, Justice Benjamin Cardozo delivered a legal premise which, along with the others, has profoundly shaped American health-care jurisprudence ever since: "Every human being of adult years and sound mind has a right to determine what shall be done with his own body."[13]

Theresa (Terri) Schiavo

Floridian Terri Schiavo was twenty-six years old when she experienced a medical anomaly that contributed to her falling onto the floor of her home in cardiac arrest. Nancy Cruzan was twenty-six at the time of her Missouri automobile accident. Terri's unfortunate collapse occurred on February 23, 1990, somewhat similarly to that of twenty-one-year-old Karen Ann Quinlan in New Jersey in 1975. Before their deaths, Quinlan remained in the vegetative state for ten years, Cruzan for almost eight years, and Schiavo for more than fifteen years. Consistently, our position has been applicable to each of these cases: If there is clear and convincing evidence of patient preference, the wishes of the patient should prevail. In the absence of patient preferences, the court appointed surrogate should be free to act in what is perceived to be in the patient's best interest at the time an end-of-life decision is required.

Terri's request on matters such as those involving herself had been earlier expressed to her husband, Michael. Etched on Terri Schiavo's tombstone are words placed there by Michael, echoing the ones on the headstone of Nancy Cruzan[14]:

Theresa Marie Schiavo
Beloved Wife
Born December 3, 1963
Departed this Earth / February 23, 1990
At peace March 31, 2005
I Kept My Promise

Michael Schiavo, the legally appointed surrogate in this case, and his wife's attending physician felt that meaningful life for her had ended years before death was finally declared. Michael added the last phrase, "I kept my promise," in reference to the fact that early in their marriage he and Terri discussed medical eventualities which in fact they later were to experience. They had concluded that neither would want to be left in a horribly debilitated condition on life-support systems, if placed there by disease or accident. Michael remained adamant to the end that he had an obligation, as Terri's legal surrogate, to implement what he knew to be her wishes. Physician-ethicist Timothy Quill notes that, "After three years of trying traditional and experimental therapies, Mr. Schiavo accepted the neurologists' diagnosis of an irreversible persistent vegetative state .... recalling prior statements she had made, such as 'I don't want to be kept alive on a machine.' "[15]

None of these three unfortunate individuals, Quinlan, Cruzan and Schiavo, had executed advance directives, which is hardly unusual since their youthful ages normally precluded thoughts that their health would soon be terribly compromised. However, all three engaged in meaningful conversations on end-of-life issues with family and friends at significant points prior to their respective demise. That dialogue proved to be crucial in each of the cases when a plethora of issues began to cloud the subsequent bedside decision, whether or not to withhold or to withdraw treatment. Terri's pronouncements to that end had been made not only to her husband Michael, but also to his brother Scott and his wife Joan on separate occasions. Sworn testimonies in trial show that:

> The court does find that Terri Schiavo did make statements which are credible and reliable with regard to her intention given the situation at hand. . . . Statements which Terri Schiavo made which do support the relief sought by her surrogate (Petitioner/Guardian) include statements to him prompted by her grandmother being in intensive care that if she ever were a burden she would not want to live like that. Additionally, statements made to Michael Schiavo which were prompted by something on television regarding people on life support that she would not want life like that also reflect her intention in this particular situation. Also the statements she made in the presence of Scott Schiavo at the funeral luncheon for his grandmother that 'if I ever go like that just let me go. Don't leave me there. I don't want to be kept alive on a machine,' and to Joan Schiavo following a television movie in which a man following an accident was in a coma to the effect that she wanted it stated in her will that she would want the tubes and everything taken out if that ever happened to her are likewise reflective of this intent. The court specifically finds that these statements are Terri Schiavo's oral declarations concerning her intention as to what she would want done under the present circumstances and the testimony regarding such oral declaration is reliable, is credible and rises to the level of clear and convincing evidence to this court.[16]

Autonomy, we have concluded repeatedly, is the right to self-determination, and is a quintessential legal principle of English common law and a bedrock of American jurisprudence. Medical autonomy, initially critical in the much earlier cases of Botsford, Mohr, and Schloendorf, was upheld by the U.S. Supreme Court in the 1990 Cruzan decision and almost simultaneously affirmed by the Patient Self-determination Act in the U.S. Congress in December of 1990. Likewise, all fifty state legislatures, including Florida, already had passed their versions of the "Right to Natural Death" acts.

Additionally, the Florida State Supreme Court in the Guardianship (surrogate) Case of Browning versus Herbert had declared in 1990, "Thus we begin with the premise that everyone has a fundamental right to the sole control of his or her person. . . . Recognizing that one has the inherent right to make choices about medical treatment, we necessarily conclude that this right encompasses all medical choices."[17] It was therefore surprising to this author and many in the field of health law and ethics that legal surrogate Michael Schiavo's 1998 petition to a Florida court for the removal of Terri's feeding tube would result in such emotional and irrational, legal, social, theological, political turmoil and cultural death denial over the next seven years. Legal/ethics authority George Annas is one of those professionals who seemed rather astonished by the unexpected outcomes emanating from this case and cites other professional groups who were as well:

> Since Ms. Schiavo was in a medical and legal situation almost identical to those of two of the most well-known patients in medical jurisprudence, Karen Ann Quinlan and Nancy Cruzan, there must be something about cases like theirs that defies simple solutions, whether medical or legal. In this sense the case of Terri Schiavo provides an opportunity to examine issues that most lawyers, bio-ethicists, and physicians believed were well settled.[18]

The gastric tube, through which liquid nutrients were channeled into Terri's stomach, kept her vegetating for fifteen years after its insertion in 1990. The U.S. Supreme Court, in the 1990 Cruzan case had opined that such feeding tubes were medical treatment and therefore could be refused or withdrawn by patients and/or their surrogates who might opt for hospice-type palliative care only. Robert M. Fine, M.D. expresses uneasiness at the widespread public failure to interpret the issues involved in this case:

> I was startled by the degree of misunderstanding about different types of brain injury and by more than a few misstatements about the medical facts of the case. Mrs. Schiavo was described at various times as comatose, brain dead, vegetative, minimally conscious, locked in, and disabled. These are mutually exclusive conditions. This failure of the media, politicians, and even some physicians who should know better to accurately describe Mrs. Schiavo's medical condition was particularly disturbing, because good medical ethics begins not with the discipline of ethics but with good clinical medicine.[19]

One fundamental difference in the Schiavo case, as opposed to Quinlan and Cruzan, was the fierce internal family struggle that ensued when the parents of Terri Schiavo, Robert and Mary Schindler, became alienated from Terri's husband, Michael. Most accounts indicate that, initially, there was harmony among the in-laws. On June 18, 1990, a Florida court appointed Michael Schiavo as Terri's legal guardian and surrogate, with no apparent objection on the part of the Schindlers.[20] Two years later, Terri received $250,000 in a non-adjudicated settlement. Several months later, Michael sued one of Terri's physicians in a malpractice case and was, due to the accident, awarded $750,000 for her care and $300,000 personal loss for himself (The State of Missouri Medicaid program had expended about $130,000 per year for the cost of Nancy Cruzan's persistent vegetative care for almost eight years).

Court records indicate that the Terri Schiavo hospitalization trust fund was devotedly and appropriately managed by her husband.[21] However, in 1993, discord erupted between the Schindlers and Michael relative to the parents' dissatisfaction regarding Terri's care, as well as apparent concern for money issues.[22] On July 29, 1993, a court denied the petition of Mary and Bob Schindler that Michael Schiavo be dismissed as Terri's guardian and surrogate.[23]

From 1993 until the request for feeding tube removal in May of 1998, nothing occurred that had significant legal impact on the Schiavo case unless one wants to argue that Michael's growing relationship with another woman, repugnant to some, accepted by others, might be reason enough for him to be stripped of his right to serve as Terri's legal surrogate. The courts consistently held, however, that Michael was Terri's legal surrogate and could serve as her guardian until, much later, her feeding tube was permanently removed on March 18, 2005, by order of Florida Circuit Court (Probate Division) Judge George W. Greer after years of legal maneuvering. The day before, on March 17, 2005, a petition to the U.S. Supreme Court filed by the Schindlers to block the removal of Terri's feeding tube was denied.[24] The next day, an attempt by the U.S. House of Representatives and the U.S. Senate failed also. Terri died thirteen days later on March 31, 2005.[25] Evidence that Terri had made her health-care wishes known to Michael and other witnesses, was deemed by Judge Greer to be clear and convincing, similar to that presented in the Quinlan and Cruzan cases.

Much earlier, in May of 1998, legal surrogate Michael Schiavo's lawyer initially filed a petition on his behalf in Judge Greer's court to have the physicians remove Terri's feeding tube. That it took seven years to adjudicate the final removal of the feeding tube is a matter of grave concern when considering the legal maxim "Justice Delayed Is Justice Denied." It should be noted, as the courts did, that Michael Schiavo, as legal surrogate since June 1990, appeared to be very patient and caring through eight years at that point in the clinical medical maintenance of Terri.[26] She struggled through the sleep/wake cycles of the persistent vegetative state, with no medical indication whatsoever of having recovered from her permanently impaired lack of cognition.

On February 11, 2000, a legal and political firestorm, which raged nationwide for five years, was initiated in that same court when Judge Greer ruled, commensurate with findings in other state jurisdictions and the U.S. Supreme Court, that Terri's feeding tube could legally be removed. My view is that Judge Greer had his finger on the pulse of correct legal process based on solid medical indications. In contrast, there were many others nationwide who appeared to be swayed by political and religious posturing, several flawed medical opinions, and intense but misguided state and federal government reaction and initiatives.

Judge Greer, for almost two years, carefully heard the medical, moral, and legal arguments for the removal of Terri Schiavo's feeding tube. Then, I contend, he turned to legal precedence that would give credence to the support of such arguments, and he made his judgment on the legal maxim of stare decisis, "the doctrine that legal principles of law serving as the basis for a court's decision are valid for subsequent cases involving substantially the same facts."[27] Judge Greer's view was, and this author concurs, that his decision should have brought the issue to a conclusion.

On April 24, 2001, Terri's gastric tube was initially removed. Legal appeals twice forced the reinsertion of the tube, and twice more over the years precipitated its removal. In the meantime, in excess of ninety courtroom appeals, rejections, petitions, reverses, stays, declinations, including state and federal legislative efforts over a five-year period of legal maneuvering, failed to halt the final medical intervention to remove the tube providing artificial nutrition and hydration.[28] Medical indications throughout, as well as the autopsy afterwards, overwhelmingly demonstrated that Schiavo was blind, experienced severe neocortical brain damage, and was not cognizant of the initial feeding tube placement or anything else before or thereafter.

Earlier, on August 11, 2001, Mary and Bob Schindler released a video that shows Terri sitting up in a hospital bed. With her non-focusing eyes wide open, the Schindler's, in abject denial, claimed that she was trying to communicate with them or others at the bedside. It was this one deceptive image, aptly described by many as "video diagnosis," which was displayed repeatedly on television screens and in newspapers and magazines for several years, creating a classic worldwide culture of death denial and judgment by numerous political, journalistic, and ecclesiastical professionals and great numbers in the lay public.

One highly profiled senator, Rick Santorum from Pennsylvania, likened pulling Schiavo's feeding tube to an "execution!'"[29] Then he stated on another occasion, "Terri Schiavo was given a death sentence and passed away without due process."[30] Other senators were "vowing to hold the judiciary system responsible for rulings in this case that some believe were tantamount to murder."[31] House Majority Leader Tom Delay exclaimed, "This loss happened because our legal system did not protect the people who need protection the most, and that will change."[32] The effusive video representation had given rise to near hysteria in the state legislature and governor's mansion of Florida, in the executive offices and halls of Congress in Washington, and among individuals in the media and general public. Politics, not medical science or the law, was fueling the mania.

The Florida state legislature on October 15, 2003, unwisely passed a bill, signed by Governor Jeb Bush, called "Terri's Law," ordering the replacement of the feeding tube that had been removed. This bill was ruled unconstitutional by a Florida judge and later by that state's Supreme Court. The U.S. Supreme Court refused to hear the Schindler's appeal. A similar version of "Terri's Law" was later passed in the U.S. House and Senate and signed near 1:00 a.m. on March 21, 2005, by President George W. Bush, who returned from a vacation in Texas for that sole purpose. With terse candor, lawyer/ethicist, George Annas observed later,

> For the first time in the history of the United States, Congress met in a special session emergency session on Sunday, March 20, to pass legislation aimed at the medical care of one patient—Terri Schiavo. . . . The brief debate on this bill in the House of Representatives (there were no hearings in either chamber and no debate at all in the U.S. Senate) was noted primarily for its uninformed and frenetic rhetoric. It was covered live on television by C-Span.[33]

Constitutionally it was a failed effort! Many across a broad and varied spectrum did not understand why! They simply did not grasp the medical indication that Terri Schiavo was a "vegetable." Her lower brain stem was functioning—her agitated body periodically stirred—but cognitively she was non-functional—her eyes were open, but she saw no one or no thing—her *person* was not present—she was, in fact, neocortically devastated as court records affirm, but her body was being kept alive by artificial nutrition and hydration flowing into her stomach through a plastic tube. Court documents state:

> Turning to the medical issues of the case, the court finds beyond all doubt that Theresa Marie Schiavo is in a persistent vegetative state or the same is defined by Florida Statutes Section 765.101 (12) per the specific testimony of Dr. James Barnhill and corroborated by Dr. Vincent Gambone. The medical evidence before the court conclusively establishes that she has no hope of ever regaining consciousness and therefore capacity, and that without the feeding tube she will die in seven to fourteen days. The un-rebutted medical testimony before this court is that such death will be painless. . . . But the overwhelming credible evidence is that Terri Schiavo has been totally unresponsive since lapsing into the coma almost ten years ago, that her movements are reflexive and predicated on brain stem activity alone, that she suffers from severe structural brain damage and to a large extent her brain has been replaced by spinal fluid.[34]

The video tape of Terri underscores the beguiling nature of the persistent vegetative state with its sleep-wake cycles. If that particular image were all the evidence that one had in responding to the Schiavo situation, it is understandable that otherwise competent professionals in the news media, in politics, in religion, and the rank and file of the public sector, could be misled en masse. But there was more, much more clinically validating information, if only those of knee-jerk response and intractable denial would have bothered to look for it or ask for it. It was upon this clinical medical data that the case was morally, legally, and appropriately adjudicated. A preponderance of neurological medical data combined with expertise from mainstream clinicians in ethics and law, had concluded many times through the preceding years that withdrawal of nutrition and hydration from a person in such a persistent vegetative state as Terri is an appropriate medical procedure—emphatically so when it is consistent with the wishes of the patient, expressed in advance through her surrogate. With feeding tube permanently withdrawn on March 18, 2005, therefore, Terri Schiavo was finally allowed a natural dying process and succumbed to a painless death from dehydration on March 31, 2005.

Thus, it appears that the primary retardant in the Terri Shiavo legal procedures was the inability of the persons whom she had loved most, her husband and her parents, to reconcile their differences. Sadly, the rancor continued through the clinical removal of Terri's feeding tube, the determination of death, and the interment of her cremains. The Schindlers were prevented participation in the interment by Michael Schiavo, due to his fear of their disruption. An April 1, 2005, newspaper article reported the account of a separate Memorial Celebration of Life, an interdenominational service attended by Terri's family and friends and 400 supporters of their cause. Father Terry Gensemer, a Roman Catholic priest, one of the liturgists in the memorial said, "Terri was murdered by the System, by legalism, and by the System's Culture of Death."[35]

The familial and societal alienation no doubt continues to this day, intrudes on the process of grief rehabilitation, and locks Terri's family into a continuing and exhausting netherworld journey. The loss of a loved one is devastating under any circumstance, but such a deprivation in the midst of conflicting medical, moral, and legal values makes a bad situation worse, magnifies grief, and prevents closure. No one should want to be judgmental or to benefit at the expense of others, but the value of seeking conciliation and closure can be learned from the Schiavo case and its years of struggle at the bedside and in the courts.

Contrastingly, twenty-six years ago, in March of 1983, television, newspapers, and professional journals shared the story of Paul E. Brophy, a forty-nine-year-old Boston firefighter who suffered a basilar artery bifurcation aneurism, which subsequently destroyed much of his mid brain. With lower-brain stem support, his cardio-respiratory system continued to function, though he was left permanently in a vegetative state. Two years later, in May of 1985, his wife petitioned a probate court in Dedham, Massachusetts, to have his feeding and hydration tube discontinued. As an emergency firefighter, Brophy had on several occasions seen hapless victims purportedly *saved* through artificial medical procedures, only to linger on life-support systems indefinitely. Earlier discussions with his family had made it clear that he did not wish to be kept alive by such procedures, if the situation ever presented itself.

The probate judge in Dedham, David H. Kopelman, held an eight-day trial to determine whether his earlier expressed wish should be granted on the legal principle of autonomy, that the right to die is an integral part of one's right to control his own destiny. Such an opinion had similarly been expressed by Brophy's wife and his Roman Catholic priest. After the eight-day hearing of professional legal, medical, and ethical testimony, the judge ruled that even though the patient's wishes were clear, the state could not condone the removal of the nasogastric tube. His ruling favored what he perceived at that time was a more significant state interest, the preservation of human life. "It is ethically inappropriate to cause the preventable death of Brophy by the deliberate denial of food and water, which can be provided to him in a nonintrusive manner which causes no pain and suffering, irrespective of the substituted judgment of the patient.[36]

However, on February 14, 1986, in a landmark ruling the Supreme Judicial Court of Massachusetts, by a five-to-four vote reversed the decision of the lower court. It ruled that artificial feeding, like artificial respiration, was a medical means of life support that could be removed based on the legal principal of "Substituted Judgment":

> In 1977 the Supreme Court of Massachusetts held in the *Saikewicz* case that decisions to withhold or withdraw life—prolonging treatment from terminally ill, incompetent patients must be made according to the test of "substituted judgment." Substituted judgment requires that surrogate decision makers act in accordance with the patient's wishes as they were expressed when the patient was competent. Further legal backing for the standard of substituted judgment came in *Brophy v. New England Sinai Hospital, Inc.* In Brophy, the Supreme Judicial Court of Massachusetts authorized removal of the artificial feeding tube from an incompetent patient in a persistent vegetative state. It held that the "substituted judgment" of an incompetent person in a persistent

vegetative state to refuse artificially administered sustenance must be honored.[37]

Having been in an irreversible coma for two years, the initial probate court petition suing for relief was filed on February 6, 1985. On February 14, 1986, one year and eight days later with the Massachusetts higher court decision, the legal process was over—in stark contrast to the elongated process suffered in the Schiavo case and its distorted efforts to nullify reasonable judicial decisions and to replace them with resolutions springing from contrived legislative and executive governmental decrees, along with exacerbated and ill-informed public opinion.

It is ironic that the legal system, despite the efficacious decisions of Circuit Court Judge George W. Greer and the higher Florida courts, held Terri Schiavo in technological captivity as long as it did, given the fact that her husband, Michael, earlier had been acknowledged by the courts to be her legal surrogate. An article in the highly respected journal, *Annals of Internal Medicine,* concludes: "In our opinion the law did not fail Terri Schiavo. In fact, no-end-of life guardianship case in U.S. history has generated as much high quality evidence, juridical attention, or legal scrutiny as the Terri Schiavo case."[38]

I agree essentially with these authors about the preponderance of medical data supporting Judge Greer's decision, though feeling the need to issue a moral and legal caveat. What followed Judge Greer's initial ruling that Terri's feeding tube be removed was arguably a sad period of legal maneuvering and inability of all involved to deliver timely closure and justice without excessive delay. Dr. Timothy Quill raises the essential question:

> How can it be that medicine, ethics, law, and family could work so poorly together in meeting the needs of this woman who was left in a persistent state after having a cardiac arrest? . . . sustained by artificial hydration and nutrition through a feeding tube for 15 years.[39]

Dr. Quill's question arguably suggests that something else must have been fomenting there, issues that continue to fester, unresolved. George Annas, apparently in agreement with Quill, retrospectively referred to the case and related it to a "Culture of Life," articulated by former President George W. Bush and which Annas believes exists in the politics of contemporary society. At the Terri Schiavo memorial service, the liturgist priest referred to "the System and a Culture of Death," which presumably ensnares us. Agreeing with Annas on his "death perspective," an additional view of my own centers on the Schiavo case and cites it and other cases occurring before and after it as operating in a "Culture of Death Denial."

In speaking to the American Bar Association, Chief Justice Warren E. Burger sounded the alarm in 1970 concerning delay in the U.S. court systems and its ramification for the delivery of justice:

> A sense of confidence in the courts is essential to maintain the fabric of ordered liberty for a free people and three things could destroy that confidence and do incalculable damage to society: that people come to believe that inefficiency and delay will drain even a just judgment of its value; that people who have long been exploited in the smaller transactions of daily life come to believe that courts cannot vindicate their legal rights from fraud and over reaching; that people come to believe the law—in the larger sense-cannot fulfill its primary function to protect them and their families in their homes, at their work, and on the public streets.[40]

That there is still-urgent need for our larger national community to learn from these dire situations was evidenced, I contend, in the widespread societal misunderstanding of the basic diagnosis of and prognosis for the persistent vegetative state. Given the preponderance of legal precedence, if the law cannot resolve the issues in a reasonable period of time when a family and large portions of a nation disagree with a court verdict, at the very least it falters and there must be explanations for the hesitations and delays. The answers, perhaps, may be found in focusing on current definitions of death and the use of the terms *Culture of Life*, *Culture of Death*, and

Culture of Death Denial, along with their impact on the delay of justice.

Chapter XI

Implications for Denial of Justice At the End of Life

Several widely accepted moral principles which have emanated from the foregoing health-care cases are: the individual's right to autonomy, to self-determination, to privacy, and to justice—commensurate with the right to refuse, withhold, and withdraw from medical treatment. A major concern at this juncture, albeit, is that autonomy devoid of justice is an empty vessel and that justice delayed is justice denied. Professor Maguire exclaims that "justice is the key":

> As Aristotle said, it is **justice** that holds the city together. Without it, society disintegrates. All laws are efforts to do justice and governments are legitimate only inasmuch as they serve justice. 'An un-just law is no law at all'—*lex mala lex nulla.* . . . It's our starter response to what persons are worth. If we do not give people justice, we have declared them worthless and we might as well incinerate them as Hitler did to those he found worthless.[1]

In an earlier chapter, we exulted in examples of self-determination in Pericles' ancient Greece and Thomas Jefferson's early America. Contrasting renderings of history, however, reveal these respective political undertakings to be huge moral contradictions, which ironically portended the denial of justice. Political, economic, and social efforts toward equal distribution of unrestrained rights were pitted against historical realities that show that "only 43,000 elites of ancient Athens-Attica population of 315,000" were considered qualified to participate in the noble experiment of Pericles, according to historian Will Durant. "All of the 115,000 slaves of Attica, all women, nearly all workingmen, all of the 28,500 'metics' or resident aliens, and consequently a great part of the trading class, are excluded from the franchise."[2] There is hardly the need to argue that this was a classic example of justice denied to many and what might be called "esoteric justice," fairness only for the few!

Thomas Jefferson's eloquent declaration of the right to self-determination in 1776 and the emergent U.S. Constitution, did not demonstrate the cause of justice for Native Americans, women, and slaves any better than did elite counterparts in ancient Greece, though historian Howard Zinn states with mitigation, "To say that the Declaration of Independence, even by its own language, was limited to life liberty and happiness for white males, is not to denounce the makers and signers of the Declaration for holding the ideas expected of privileged males of the eighteenth century."[3] Perhaps one can say that, at the least, the Declaration of Independence was an initial clang on the bell of liberty and a hammer on the anvil of justice. The subsequent constitution was and is an incremental work in progress. There is poetic irony in the current display in Philadelphia of the Liberty Bell with a significant crack in it and currently imaged on our postage stamps, a bell that does not always ring *perfectly* true, not then—not now.

For Native American Indians, the period that followed the Declaration of 1776 was 150 years of slaughter, broken treaties, and delayed social, economic, and political justice, until the Indian Citizenship Act of 1924 was passed by Congress, procrastination which continues in part to the present day. As for African Americans, "The United States government's support of slavery," reports Zinn, "was based on an overpowering practicality. In 1790, a thousand tons of cotton were being produced every year in the South. By 1860, it was a million tons. In the same period, 500,000, slaves grew to 4 million."[4] Slaves were freed in the 11 Southern States of the Confederacy by the Emancipation Proclamation of President Lincoln on January 1, 1863, in the midst of the Civil War. Abolition of slavery was proposed by Lincoln and some in Congress on January 31, 1865. The President was mortally wounded on April 14th of that year and died on April 15th. The more comprehensive Abolition of Slavery Act was ratified by congress on December 6, 1865. Most men (exclusive of Native Americans), regardless of race, color, or previous condition of servitude were granted the right to vote, when the 15th Amendment to the Constitution was ratified on February 8, 1870. Women of all colors, classes, or races were denied full participation in that proclaimed act of enfranchisement. In the aftermath of the 1776 Declaration of Independence and the Constitution which followed, women were sequestered together in a category all to themselves until they were finally granted suffrage in 1919 with the passage of the 19th Amendment. Regarding the Declaration of 1776, contemporary historian Howard Zinn writes:

> The use of the phrase 'all men are created equal' was probably not a deliberate attempt to make a statement about women. It was just that women were beyond consideration as worthy of inclusion. They were politically invisible. Though practical needs gave women a certain authority in the home, on the farm, or in occupations like midwifery, they were simply overlooked in any consideration of political rights, any notion of civic equality.[5]

In spite of the Emancipation Proclamation and Abolition, significant efforts to disenfranchise former slaves and all African Americans continued into the twentieth century throughout the southern states by way of Jim Crow laws, segregation, and the poll tax. Such laws effectively kept poor Blacks in the South from casting their vote for many decades, into the latter part of the twentieth century. When I moved to Alabama in 1963 with my wife and children, the poll tax was still in place, and for the privilege of voting in the 1964 presidential election, my wife and I each paid a two-dollar poll tax. Though vexed by the law, we had the money and reluctantly paid it, but many poor rural and inner-city Blacks did not. On April 16, 1963, Martin Luther King, Jr., released his famous "Letter From Birmingham Jail," written in response to White Birmingham ministers who were calling upon him to cease and desist with civil rights demonstrations in the city, relative not only to voting restrictions upon Blacks but to all segregation and discrimination:

> We know through painful experience that freedom is never voluntarily given by the oppressor: it must be demanded by the oppressed. I have yet to engage in a direct-action campaign that was "well timed" in the view of those who have not suffered unduly from the disease of segregation. For years now I have heard the

word 'Wait!' It rings in the ear of every Negro with piercing familiarity. This 'Wait' has almost always meant 'Never.' We must come to see, with one of our distinguished jurists, that 'justice too long delayed is justice denied.'[6]

Finally, the Supreme Court in 1966 held that a tax levied for the privilege of voting was unconstitutional. The last four states to fall seriatim under federal mandate were Texas, Alabama, Virginia, and Mississippi. Justice, related to suffrage, was becoming far more achievable for many in the U.S.A.

Justice has a most vital role to play in the ethical and moral delivery of health care but, as has been shown, justice oftentimes presents incrementally, in small bytes. It is a legal maxim that the wheels of justice grind slowly but exceedingly fine; at other times, for some, they may not grind at all. In reflecting on the three sides of justice, Maquire states, "We relate on a one-to-one basis (commutative justice), individuals relate to the social whole (social justice); and the representatives of the social whole relate back to individuals (distributive justice)."[7]

In the present day health-care situation, justice is the acknowledgement that clinical medical ethics and moral values should be critical components of the policies and procedures that take place within the context of shared values, equal distribution of resources, and clinical responsibility—it shuns individualism and isolationism and radiates social and relational values—it lifts up the values of the patient, the physician, the hospital and its professional staff, and the values and laws of the community. Such is the current challenge to health-care ethics and morality, as the cases of Quinlan, Cruzan, Brophy, and Schiavo have demonstrated, and how they incrementally advanced the causes of autonomy and justice.

As noted in the preceding chapter, however, legal analyst and ethicist George Annas was recognizably chagrined by the legislative proceedings and political fallout from the Terri Schiavo case. He takes umbrage at the views expressed by President George Bush who flew back to Washington from vacation in Texas to sign the special congressional efforts relative to Schiavo. After signing the hasty and scantily debated legislation, Bush made reference to a "culture of life":

> The case of Terri Schiavo raises complex issues. . . . Those who live at the mercy of others deserve our special care and concern. It should be our goal as a nation to build a culture of life, where all Americans are valued, welcomed, and protected—and that culture of life must extend to individuals with disabilities.[8]

President Bush expresses here a view that is held in this country by Americans on the far right of the social, religious, and political spectrum in regard to issues at the end of life, articulated by Pope John Paul II on March 25, 1995, in a papal encyclical. This culture of life within the beginning-of-life perspective takes sanctity of life in its larval stage to its absolutist perspective as well. Potential life, represented by the zygote, embryo, and fetus is invariably seen by these enthusiasts as having value disproportionate to the physical and psychological well-being of the mother and significant others. In their view, it also has value beyond every other moral consideration where existing *life* is often *pitted* against *life* in its beginning stages—medical indications of physical or mental deformity, conception as a result of rape or incest, or the socio-economic and psychological condition of the individual and the family, to mention several. Dissenting Catholic moral theologian Charles Curran takes exception to the papal encyclical and appears to be supportive of the views of this author on this issue:

> In conflict situations the life of the fetus may be taken to save the life of the mother. Even the Catholic tradition in the question of unjust aggression permitted the killing of the aggressor to save chastity or material goods of great value. Thus in conflict situations I would allow abortion to save human life. This would obviously include grave but real threats to the psychological health of the woman and could also include other values of a socio-economic nature in extreme situations.[9]

At the other extremity, aggressive end-of-life treatment is likely to be extended far beyond reasonable scientific evidence that the burdens of treatment excessively outweigh the benefits of treatment. This was demonstrated earlier in the Quinlan family "faith-related" reluctance to have the feeding tube removed during her ten years of persistent vegetative state, as well as in the Terri Schiavo case, which exacerbated Bush's use of the term "culture of life." I would argue that, at *both ends* of the spectrum, justice is regularly denied by this over-reaching culturalization of life.

This tunnel vision approach sharply limits the scope of moral decision making by shutting out all other perspectives at the top, bottom, and on all sides of the issue as if one were looking through a tube. The larger picture is missed, at times intentionally, for to broaden the view would be to destroy the priority. The search for moral truth, on the other hand, includes all things on the periphery as well as at the center—includes many facets not just one. Single-issue exponents may be sharply focused on their mission, but in the process often do violence to the larger truth, which is that "pro choice" adherents may have equal concern about the "sanctity and sacredness of life" along with intransigent oppositionists at the other extremity.

"Pro-lifers," "right-to-lifers," and "sanctity of lifers," invariably raise the spectra of holocaust when alternative rights of selectivity and choice are advocated. They point to the medical atrocities perpetrated by the Nazis in Germany during the nineteen-thirties and early forties and draw analogies of evil and murder, which are applied to beginning-of-life and end-of-life issues in general. Obviously the new technologies and concurrently new ethical dilemmas posed by every advance of science cannot be ignored. That is precisely what bio-medical ethics is all about, but one must not be stampeded to the extremes by flawed arguments and irrational solutions. Enthusiasm for only a portion of the truth should not be allowed to crowd out the sum total of truth, nor must we allow the conscience and freedom of the individual to be denied.

"Erring on the side of life in this context often results in violating a person's body and human dignity in a way few would want for themselves," wrote George Annas, in his article concerning the end-of-life Schiavo case. Then he states "In such situations, erring on the side of liberty—specifically the patient's right to decide on treatment—is more consistent with American values and our constitutional traditions." Finally, as a point of reference, Annas cites a 1977 Massachusetts Supreme Judicial Court decision of a similar case:

> The constitutional right to privacy, as we conceive it, is an expression of the sanctity of individual free choice and self-determination as fundamental constituents of life. The value of life as so perceived is lessened not by a decision to refuse treatment, but by the failure to allow a competent human being the right of choice.[10]

When the Roman Catholic priest at the Schindler family memorial service for Terri Schiavo, referred to the "system and the culture of death," he was placing in one huge bucket all of the pronouncements of those on the political, social, and Protestant Christian religion's extreme right, along with most of the Roman bishops, the Pope, and anyone who adheres to the principle of "culture of life" at all cost. One source in simple terms, defines the principle, "It is described by its proponents as a philosophy that human life, at all stages from conception through natural death, is sacred. As such, a 'culture of life' is claimed to be opposed to practices seen by its proponents as destructive to life." There is an assumption that any health-care procedure that threatens a thoroughgoing acceptance of the maxim "culture of life" is of the culture of death, such as distrust of government, conspiracy theories, contemporary death panels, withholding/withdrawing care, contraceptives, and the like.

The priest during the Terri Schiavo memorial affixed the "Death Culture" label upon the physicians, judges, theologians, and ethicists involved in the end-of-life withdrawal of treatment and conclusion of the Schiavo case upon her death in 2005. Earlier, Catholic moral theologian William May in 2001, pursuing beginning-of-life issues, was applying the same condemnatory label onto any Roman Catholic and all others who were resorting to "contraception" instead of periodic abstinence and the "rhythm of the cycle" method of birth control. In a sweeping constriction of personal freedom and denial of individual autonomy, he writes in the journal *Faith* "It is for this reason that the recourse to the rhythm of the cycle is the 'gateway' to the culture of life, just as its opposite, *contraception,* is the gateway to the culture of death."[11]

Fast forwarding to the current era, Brian Murphy, within an Associated Press article on March 15, 2013 (The Tennessean), reflects on theological and social views of newly elected Pope Francis reiterating pronouncements of the church leadership expressed a decade and a half earlier:

> There is no doubt about Frances' traditional groundings. He has spoken out resolutely in support of central Catholic tenants, echoing the words of Pope John Paul II to call abortion and contraception part of a 'culture of death' and showing no public tolerance for homosexuality. In fights against plans in Argentina to legalize same-sex marriages, he described such unions as 'a scheme to destroy God's plan.'

Admittedly, M. Gregg Bloche, M.D., J.D. presents a mitigating perspective on the issue of delay, with which we have been contending. He argues that the vast majority of end-of-life and persistent-vegetative-state case disagreements are currently settled at the bedside without resort to action in the civil courts.

> End-of-life questions are almost always resolved in the private sphere, by patients, their physicians, and their family members, working with nurses, social workers, and members of the clergy. In tens of thousands of cases each year, patients and families handle catastrophic illness or injury without going to court. They do so with unsung courage, in the face of fear, anguish, and sometimes bitterness. . . . Anger and denial are common, especially when relationships were conflict-ridden beforehand. What is remarkable, given the intensity of the feelings at stake, is how rarely such conflicts make their way to court.[12]

Dr. Bloche's article is a convincing reminder that clinical decision making on neocortical issues is functioning at least with minimally reasonable levels of success and that the situation could perhaps be a great deal worse than presently exists. He appears to admit though, and rightly so, that the bedside negotiations are fraught with "bitterness, anger and denial," differences that cloud the issues, and obviously delay withdrawals of technological support, especially in persistent vegetative cases.

Therefore, one must ask, could the clinical environment in many instances be made more congenial and specific and less complex? I am advocating that that it could be! The "Culture of Life-Culture of Death" syndrome remains a disconcerting subliminal force operating discretely below the threshold of consciousness of many in this country—a major cause of the fear, anguish, bitterness, denial, and resultant indecision to which Dr. Bloche refers. Without a clear definition of how neocortical disaster destroys the existence of the *person* while the *breathing corpse* is maintained vegetatively, the lay public and many professionals will continue in what Annas has called a "Culture of Life," what the priest has called a "Culture of Death," and what I have called a "Culture of Death Denial."

Aristotle's observation in moral discourse is germane: "Shall we not, like archers who have a mark to aim at, be more likely to hit upon what is right?"[13] The Christian New Testament uses a similar metaphor: "It is the same with lifeless instruments that produce sound, such as the flute or the harp. If they do not give distinct notes, how will anyone know what is being played. And if the bugle gives an indistinct sound, who will get ready for battle?"[14]

Is it not plausible to argue that the surrogates and families of neocortically devastated patients are more likely to accept the fact that a loved one is in an irreversibly hopeless state if there were a clear technologically driven process of neocortical *definition* of death—along with the concurrent *determination* of whole-brain death? After all, Quinlan had lain in a vegetative state for ten years, Cruzan for almost eight years, and Schiavo for fifteen years.

The loved ones of Talyor Coleman, within the time frame of thirty-six hours, had to accept the fact that EEG technology unequivocally supported the diagnosis of death by Whole-Brain criteria. There was no perceived need for negotiation between the Coleman family and professional caregivers in behalf of Taylor Coleman, except at the level of transplantation. In turn, they stood by while their still-breathing son on life supports was transported to another department within Vanderbilt Medical Center where his kidneys were removed for transplantation. The respirator supporting his beating heart was then removed and, within seconds, his heart stopped beating and he was pronounced dead. Such a scenario is being replayed again and again in a great many hospitals in this country every day and, in every case, is deemed by our society to be perfectly legal, moral, and acceptable clinical procedure.

In similar situations, thousands of persons each year stand at the bedside of loved ones who lie in persistent vegetative states for indeterminable periods of time. Positron Emission Tomography (PET) scans and similar technologies can do for PVS patients what EEGs did for Whole-Brain Death diagnosis, that is, *conclusively* demonstrate that the patient is in an irreversible, incurable, and non-sentient state. When the diagnosis of irreversible PVS is thus made, the average family ostensibly could respond in the manner of the Colemans. They could either suggest that body parts be allocated for someone in desperate need of them or, in the view of Professor Roland Pucetti, could say something like, "She's dead but her body is still breathing, so we're going to stop the breathing and prepare her body for burial."[15]

From a legal perspective, attorney David Smith and others in the 1984 Vanderbilt Symposium advocating a definition of neocortical death cited a number of important issues that might surface in the event that such a definition were adopted. These include broadening possibilities for research and transplantation of organs and other body parts; appropriate management of anencephalic infants born without portions of their brains intact; questions relative to wills and property; and issues related to criminal, tort, and insurance law. In summary, Professor Smith offered helpful legal assurance, as we press for needed change in how we understand and approach death in the clinical setting:

> Giving legal effect to neocortical death, does not present any special legal problems that cannot be resolved with just results."[16]
>
> Giving legal effect to neocortical death will simplify and purify the decision to end the biological existence

of a family member and assure that the right results are reached for the right reasons.[17]

Without a neocortical definition and determination of death legally in place therefore, I continue to argue that justice will remain excessively elusive for many thousands of unfortunate patients who are imprisoned by the clinical netherworld existence of persistent vegetative state, along with their grieving families awaiting closure. Furthermore, in a time of rising costs and burgeoning shortages in financial health-care resources, such delay becomes a moral travesty at the levels of social and distributive justice, along with the denial of precious organs to thousands of patients plaintively awaiting them.

Diagram of Brain

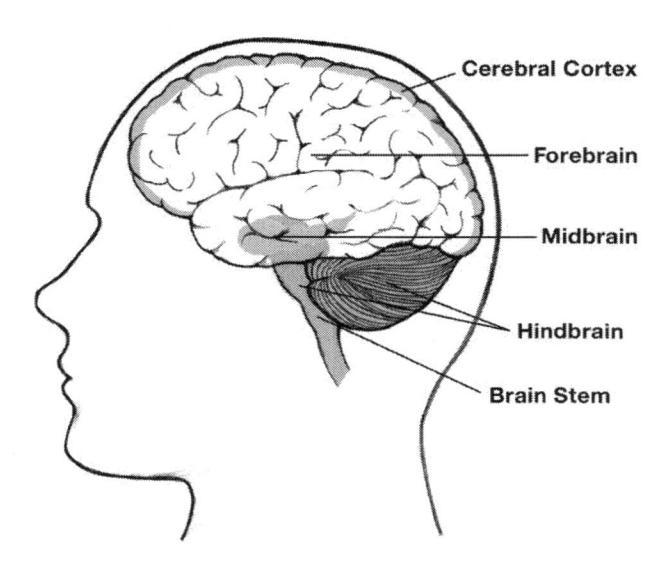

Image by Donna Pritchett

Taylor Coleman *lost* **all function** of the brain, the upper, mid, and lower regions, and within 36 hours was pronounced dead, with life supports removed after kidneys were salvaged for transplantation.

PVS patients, **Quinlan**, **Cruzan**, and **Shiavo**, *lost* **all function** of the upper brain and **Brophy** *lost* **all function** of the mid and upper brain, i.e., **cognition**, while *retaining* lower vegetative **function**. Each remained in non-sentient condition *sustained* by technology for periods ranging from 3-15 years.

Locked-in Syndrome and ALS patients *retained* **function** of the upper brain, **cognition**, but *lost* vegetative or lower **function** of the body. **Locked-in** patients immediately *lost* all lower brain, vegetative, and bodily **function** (from the nose downward. **ALS** patients gradually but definitively *lost* all vegetative **function**.

148

(Data from the National Institute of Neurological Disorders and Stroke appear in bold print below)

The brain is divided into three basic units: the forebrain, the midbrain, and the hindbrain, {For the purposes within this book, we refer to the forebrain and hindbrain as upper brain and lower brain respectively} **The forebrain** (upper) **is the largest and most highly developed part of the human brain: it consists of the cerebrum and the structures hidden beneath in the inner brain . . . the hypothalamus and thalamus. The cerebrum sits at the topmost part of the brain and is the source of intellectual activities** (cognition). **It holds your memories, allows you to plan, enables you to imagine and think. It allows you to recognize friends, read books and play games. Coating the surface of the cerebrum and the cerebellum is a vital layer of tissue the thickness of a stack of two or three dimes, It is called the cortex, from the Latin word bark. Most of the actual information processing in the brain takes place in the cerebral cortex. When people talk about "gray matter" in the brain they are talking about this thin rind. The cortex is gray . . . most other parts of the brain appear to be white.**

The midbrain is the uppermost part of the brainstem, and controls some reflex actions and is part of the circuit involved in the control of eye movements and other voluntary movements.

The hindbrain includes the upper part of the spinal cord, the brain stem, and a wrinkled ball of tissue called the cerebellum. The hind brain (lower) **controls the body's vital functions such as respiration and heart rate. The cerebellum coordinates movement and is involved in learned rote movements. When you play the piano or hit a tennis ball you are activating the cerebellum.**

Part Three

    Scientists in the National Institute of Neurological Disorders and Stroke affirm that in modes of action conversely to brain damaged PVS patients, clearly conscious and perceptive human beings can become permanently constricted within almost totally paralyzed bodies, from the nose downward.[1] This morbid condition is called "locked-in syndrome" and is detailed in the subsequent cases of John Doe I and Jean Dominique Bauby. The case of John Doe II is medically similar to locked-in syndrome and results from the syndrome Basilar Artery Bifurcation Aneurism in the midbrain.

    Scientists observe, also, that other clearly conscious and perceptive unfortunates can, over time, become *progressively* and agonizingly debilitated and subsequently unable to move arms, legs, other body parts, along with the muscular incapacity to breathe without mechanical support, ultimately to approximate physically those patients with locked-in syndrome. The condition is labeled Amyotrophic Lateral Sclerosis, or Lou Gehrig's disease, and is delineated by the cases of athlete Lou Gehrig, Jane Doe, and Nancy Gamble. As with those cases in Part Two, there is currently no cure for these tragic medical anomalies discussed in Part Three.

Chapter XII
Locked-in Syndrome
and
Basilar Artery Bifurcation Aneurism

John Doe I

In the summer of 1996, the telephone rang in the Center for Clinical Ethics of a Nashville medical center associated with a nationwide health-care system. The person on the other end of the line was a neurosurgeon on the hospital staff requesting that I, as the institutional clinical ethicist, meet him in the conference room adjacent to the medical intensive care unit. A forty-seven-year-old year old male collapsed at his workplace and was brought by EMS to the hospital emergency department in an unconscious state. After initial examination, the ER medical staff summoned the neurosurgeon to obtain additional information through imaging and other procedures.

Upon further scrutiny the patient was admitted to the hospital's critical intensive care unit. Eight or nine days later, the unfortunate individual slowly awakened and mental awareness was indicated. Progressively, over several days, he began to respond to questions posed by the physicians and nursing staff. However, he remained unable to move or communicate other than blinking his left eye in response to questions—once for "yes" and twice for "no." With a diagnosis of "locked-in syndrome" the patient was almost totally paralyzed and dependent on life support systems, including ventilator and feeding tube. This posed a significant medical dilemma and quality-of-life issue. The National Institute of Neurological Disorders and Strokes (NINDS), offers the following definition for this medical anomaly:

> Locked-in syndrome is a rare neurological disorder characterized by complete paralysis of voluntary muscles in all parts of the body except those that control eye movement. It may result from traumatic brain injury, diseases of the circulatory system, diseases that destroy the myelin sheath surrounding nerve cells, or medication overdose. Individuals with locked-in syndrome are conscious and can think and reason, but are unable to move. The disorder leaves individuals completely mute and paralyzed. Communication may be possible with blinking eye movements. . . . There is no cure for locked-in syndrome nor is there a standard course of treatment. . . . The prognosis for those with locked-in syndrome is poor. The majority of individuals do not regain function. . . . NINDS supports research on neurological disorders that can cause locked-in syndrome. The goals of this research are to find ways to prevent, treat, and cure these disorders.

As the consulting ethicist, my role in extraordinarily complex cases, when summoned by the physician of record, was to facilitate and to be a participant with him/her in a small group consultation. Initially, that conference also included the charge nurse and any other physicians integrally related to the case. The goal was to evaluate morally and legally the medical indications and a treatment or non-treatment plan to be agreed upon later at the bedside by the patient and the physician. This was especially critical because of the nature of this case and probable end-of-life ramifications. If the patient's competency were compromised by injury or disease, the treatment plan would be negotiated by a surrogate and the physician. It was vital for the professional staff members involved to be on the same page and to present a carefully delineated procedure with appropriate options. It was equally vital, later, for the patient, family, or surrogate to have a reasonable understanding of the recommended process for their making an informed decision and for giving written consent to proceed.

The 1991 Federal Self-determination Act, mentioned in a preceding chapter, was predicated on the medical, moral, and legal precept that patients have a right to participate in the clinical decisions affecting their bodies and their lives. In this particular medical center, there is a framed sign with the title in bold print at information desks, admitting offices, and waiting rooms throughout the facility, which states emphatically: **"It's Your Decision."** In addition, the sign reads: "You have the right to decide what type of medical treatment, if any, you want." It had two brief statements relative to Living Wills and Durable Power of Attorney for Health Care. Then it suggested, "You should discuss your wishes with your physician and sign these papers while you are still able."

Alongside one's right to be left alone and the right to refuse treatment, the patient has the right to be informed adequately of medical options, the risks involved in each, and the reasonable costs appertaining—a body of ethics and law that had been developing in the United States since midway in the twentieth century. This doctrine of "informed consent" was broached in the 1957 Salgo vs. Stanford University Board of Trustees case and later broadened in Canterbury vs. Spence in 1972. In the latter case, Judge Spottswood Robinson, in denial of an appeal by Dr. Spence, referred to Justice Cordozo's focus on medical self-determination in his Schloendorff decision in 1914: "Every human being of adult years and sound mind has a right to determine what shall be done with his own body. . ."[1]

The physician-patient relationship, thus, is the most logical and productive starting point for the discussion of these issues along with "advance directives." The optimum place and time for initiating these conversations is the physician's office, before the patient has a need to be admitted to a health-care facility. These discussions should be documented in the patient's medical record and any relevant conversation or advance directive may be included. Such dialogue might also embrace decisions for the donation of body parts or other pertinent concerns. However, many physician-patient relationships, as with this case of locked-in syndrome, are initiated in the midst of a medical crisis, often precluding the opportunity for advance conversations and resulting in end-of-life negotiation by strangers.

Soon after John Doe I's admission to the hospital, a married twenty-two-year-old daughter appeared, having been apprised by her father's co-workers of the fateful episode at his office. She was an only child of the patient and his former wife, so she was invited to an initial conference with the professional staff. Her conversation with the clinical staff indicated, as far as she knew, that her father had not formally executed advance directive documents—nor had he participated with any family members in dialogue about such issues. Later conversation with her mother, the patient's former spouse living in another state, produced a similar report. No one, including other family, co-workers, or friends, had any notion of what the patient's wishes might be regarding his terribly compromised state of being. According to Tennessee law and the medical center's policies and procedures, the adult daughter was therefore deemed to be in the best position to serve as the patient's decision-making surrogate, if it became necessary.

With the patient gradually becoming mentally aware, however, it was appropriate for the physician to share with him the grim prognosis, as had already been done in an earlier conference with his daughter. If any treatment decisions were to be made, the patient possibly could make them, since he was progressing cognitively. But, envision the personal horror of waking up in the clinical netherworld, to be made aware of the likelihood that more than 99 percent of one's body would never again be responsive to the signals via the brain's neurons. The impulse-conducting cells, blocked by the occlusion that devastated the brain stem, had short-circuited the body's generating and coordinating nervous system and irrevocably shut it down.

Patients or potential patients and their families soon become aware that it is the physician's role to present the diagnosis and prognosis and to suggest a treatment plan to be shared later with the mentally aware and competent patient. Furthermore, the professional staff must make it clear that whatever treatment is recommended by the physicians must conform to the established policies and procedures of the institution in which they are practicing medicine.

Diagnosis, is a derivative of two Greek words, *dia* (throughout) and *gnosis* (to know); that is, to know as thoroughly as possible. Data from the patient's in-hospital tests and examinations, along with any other accessible medical history are gathered. These data then are collated with information emanating from the physician's formal education and special clinical training relative to particular diseases and accidents—in this case, neurology/neurosurgery. Having accomplished the task of data gathering, the physician, therefore, should be prepared to share the extent of what is "known" about the patient and the anomaly affecting him and to offer a "prognosis."

Prognosis, likewise, is the fusion of two Greek words, *pro* (before) and *gnosis* (to know), that is, to know beforehand or to predict a potential outcome of the case, based on what is medically established about the disease and its actual or potential impact on the specific patient. In this instance, the medical indications forecast an end result based on phrases or percentages suggesting grimness and futility. "There is no reasonable chance of recovery," reported the neurosurgeon. "The patient has only a one percent chance of survival—even then, we do not know for how long or in what state."

Several days later, the moment for sharing more complete medical information with the patient had arrived. The daughter of the patient and the physician, the charge nurse, and I left the conference room and gathered at the patient's bedside in the intensive care unit. The patient's pastor was invited as well. Other bedside professional staff had established communication with the patient over several preceding days, as he slowly emerged from unconsciousness and stupor resulting from the brain-stem stroke. Earlier conversation about the severity of his medical condition was withheld from him by the neurosurgeon until he felt that the patient could comprehend the medical information with reasonable clarity. In this instance, the patient remained unable to move or speak and could respond to questions and comments only by blinking his left eye. He was, however, deemed to be mentally competent, able to receive and to respond to relevant information.

With candor and compassion the physician carefully explained to John Doe I the nature of the stroke he had experienced and the fragile, if not futile, state in which he was left. At the time, there were stimulating procedures that perhaps could offer short-term muscular relief and case-by-case possibilities of minimal improvement, but none to cure this primary locked-in state. Asked in several different ways if he understood the somber medical realities that now confronted him, there was one blink with his left eye for each question, indicating that he was mentally grasping the situation. When he was queried about having the life supports continued if there was no hope for improvement beyond the current state, he responded with two blinks of his left eye, indicating preference for withdrawal of treatment. When asked the same question using slightly different terms, the answer came once more with two blinks—withdrawal of life-support was preferred.

The neurosurgeon suggested to the patient, and to all persons present, that we meet back in the same room twenty-four hours later. We would go through a similar process, having pondered the ramifications of staying the course of treatment or discontinuing life supports. After all, this was the first complete medical explanation given to this patient regarding his almost total paralysis and inability to communicate beyond the use of eye movements. The attendant physician and I concluded that such a reasonable delay, to allow the patient and his daughter time to assimilate the harsh facts and to make an informed decision, was indeed medically and morally sensitive and appropriate.

On the next day at 2:00 p.m., the physician, charge nurse, case manager, and I returned the patient's room where he, his daughter, and their pastor were waiting. The neurosurgeon invited the pastor to have an initial prayer. The subsequent information-sharing process, resembling the previous one, was repeated with some derivation. The daughter requested clarification of specific medical data. Once more the patient was asked if he understood the finality of having the life supports removed on the one hand and, on the other, the arduous uncertainty of existing with incurable locked-in-syndrome. One left-eye blink indicated that he was aware. Asked once more in a slightly different way, the response was the same—he wanted to claim his right to have the life support withdrawn.

The discussion of a time line was held with the patient's daughter. As the ethics consultant, I then suggested another delay, this one for forty-eight hours, before acceding to the wishes of the patient for withdrawal. The daughter and her father had agreed earlier that they would like to have her mother, the patient's former wife if she were willing, to be there for the removal of life supports. The patient's attorney and pastor also would come and discuss with him confirmation of, or possible changes in, his estate and funeral plans. In the meantime, this final waiting period would give the patient additional opportunity to alter his treatment decision, if for any reason he were inclined to do so.

Two days later, we gathered at John Doe I's bedside for the last time. Then, as the respirator was finally removed from the patient, his family stood with their pastor outside the door to his room. Seeing the tears on the face of both the patient's daughter and his former wife, my thoughts once again were that to travel through the clinical netherworld is, indeed, a gut-wrenching, soul-searching, and often heart-breaking journey for those making complex decisions at the lowest levels of life. Retrospectively, the professional staff felt that it had striven fervently to provide this patient and his family with the appropriate information and spiritual support necessary for an informed decision, one fraught with such awesome sense of imminent futility and ultimate finality.

John Doe II[2]
Basilar Artery Bifurcation Aneurism

A prominent fifty-one-year-old attorney left his fashionable Belle Meade home early one morning for a routine jog through the neighborhood. After returning, he jumped into the shower before eating breakfast and departing for his law office in downtown Nashville. It was then that his wife heard a "thud" in the shower stall. Investigating, she found her husband slumped onto the floor and trying to talk, but with slurred speech and great difficulty. Desperately, she placed a call for 911 emergency assistance and one to her next door neighbors, a physician and his wife. The physician had already left home for surgery, but his wife rushed over to assist getting the individual onto his bed. She also telephoned a hospital emergency department to inform them of what had occurred and that emergency medical services and a patient would arrive there within minutes. She was assured that the appropriate medical staff would be summoned and waiting for them. The neighbor remained to care for the couple's three-year-old daughter who was asleep in her bedroom.

Later, they recalled that it seemed like only seconds before EMS was there to start the process of transporting the individual to a hospital. However, as the medical technicians arrived at the home, John Doe II appeared to be returning to normalcy and protested his being taken to the hospital, but his wife and the technicians prevailed—the telephone call had been made—the hospital was preparing for the patient's arrival.

The date was April 21, 1988. At some point, his wife remembered that several months earlier her husband experienced a similar episode. Momentarily, he became disoriented at home after jogging, but apparently it was short lived and he "shook it off." At the conclusion of a rigorous examination at the emergency department after this second one, a neurosurgeon initially determined that both of the experiences had the classic symptoms of a TIA (Transient Ischemic Attack.) They were going to admit the patient to the hospital, monitor his progress and, before rendering a final diagnosis, perform additional tests the next day. The National Institute of Neurological Disorders and Strokes defines TIA as follows:

> A transient ischemic attack (TIA) is a transient stroke that lasts only a few minutes. It occurs when the blood supply to part of the brain is briefly interrupted. TIA symptoms which usually occur suddenly, are similar to those of stroke but do not last as long. Most symptoms of a TIA disappear within an hour, although they may persist for up to 24 hours. Symptoms can include: numbness or weakness in the face, arm, or leg, especially one side of the body; confusion or difficulty in talking or understanding speech; trouble seeing in one or both eyes, difficulty with walking, dizziness, or loss of balance and coordination. Because there is no way to tell whether symptoms are from a TIA or an acute stroke, patients should assume that all stroke-like symptoms signal an emergency and should not wait to see if they go away.

Having been at the hospital since early morning, John Doe II's wife went home late in the afternoon to be with her three-year-old daughter. Somewhat eased, but still a bit anxious about her husband, she thanked her gracious neighbor for coming to their rescue. It was early to bed that night after an exhausting day. "All's well that ends well," she thought, after a frantic day's beginning and a sense of relief as it was concluded.

When she was awakened by a ringing telephone at 3:00 a.m., the patient's wife had reason to be alarmed. Telephone calls in the middle of the night invariably are harbingers of ominous events. A nurse was calling from the hospital. Her husband experienced significantly labored breathing and was demonstrating signs of seizure. "Code blue" had been initiated, signaling to all specified clinical staff that a patient was facing imminent crisis and potential loss of life and needed immediate emergency attention, possibly ventilator support and/or resuscitation.

Immediately, she dressed and called her next-door neighbor to stay once more with her young child. Mixed thoughts flooded her mind as she negotiated the well-lit and empty streets. She was grateful that there was little or no traffic. The usual twenty-minute trip to the hospital on the main avenue into mid town was therefore cut in half. At that hour the red and yellow traffic lights were flashing in off/on mode for easy passage. But, should she have forebodings concerning the call that awakened her so abruptly? That question essentially was answered when she arrived at her husband's room and went to his bedside. "My first impression," she recalled later, "was that he appeared to be virtually immobile and non-communicative." Then, she reached out for his hand, lifted it, only to have it fall back onto the bed at his side.

Immediately afterwards, she was asked to sign the consent form relative to an arteriogram and other tests to determine the cause and extent of this latest episode. Then there was the agonizing emotional pain and distress of those who experience the grim waiting process that typically unfolds in the clinical netherworld. The time was close to 4:00 a.m. It seemed an eternity before the neurosurgeon came to the room about 6:00 a.m. with the test results. They were not good. Her husband sustained a blockage of the basilar artery, a major channel carrying blood with its critically important oxygen to the lower backside of the brain, resulting in a brain stem stroke. She remembers, from that point onward, that the two terms (basilar artery and brain stem) were used almost interchangeably by the physicians to describe the systemic failure. They were guarded as to what collateral damage might have resulted from the insult to this vital region of the body.

"It's a critical time," the professional caregivers stated as they limited her to three brief visits a day. "And be careful about what is said when you visit," they cautioned as their demeanor changed markedly over the next forty-eight hours, from one of hopefulness to one of medical futility. Discussing with me much later her inmost recollections of those fateful experiences, John Doe II's wife was profoundly moved once more by the incongruity of the series of events. There was the initial collapse and appearance of quick recovery, the emergency room, the intensive care unit following the middle-of-the-night strokes, and the final immobility. "Here's a guy who is extremely active," she mused, as if she were reliving the events, "rides a bike, plays golf, jogs, practices law, runs for public office, and serves in the state legislature for sixteen to eighteen years; and now he can do nothing for himself."

Reverting to the past tense, she selectively gathered her memories and said, "It was very striking to be a wife/caregiver in a situation like that. I didn't want to do anything that would jeopardize what the professional caregivers were doing. He couldn't speak, but did have eye movement. Later they used the term 'locked-in'." She paused, reflected, and then continued: "At some point I realized that I could ask questions and that occasionally there would be an effort to respond with his eyes—look up for yes, down for no. So, I tried to think of everything, like reading *Sports Illustrated*, one of his favorite magazines. After several days there was little reaction. For a while, I began to ask myself, 'Is this agitating him? Am I hurting him or hindering chance of recovery?' " Such was the agonizing profundity of sitting at the bedside of a medically conflicted loved one in the clinical setting.

After two weeks into the intensive care experience, any mental alertness the patient initially displayed had diminished. MRI tests showed a series of mini strokes added to the already significant brain-stem stroke. For about ten days more in the hospital, he existed essentially in a terminal state. Near the outset of the intensive care procedures, a tracheostomy was provided by an incision (tracheotomy) for an airway directly into the windpipe, making it easier to wean the patient from a basic or more sophisticated respirator. However, he was maintained on a *demand* or *blow-by* respirator, a device in place and activated only when the patient's air needs spontaneously called for it.

John Doe II was also subsisting on a feeding tube under conditions which, ostensibly, he had rejected years earlier in an advance directive. As an attorney for a hospital, he was health-care savvy and several years earlier had executed a living will and a durable power of attorney for health care, making his wife the "attorney in fact." So, there was initial conversation concerning the removal of the feeding tube at some point. Also, the attending physicians and the patient's wife agreed that a "Do Not Resuscitate order" should be written, consistent with hospital policy and procedure in same or similar circumstances. In the event of cardiac arrest, given his terminal condition, there would be no clinical effort to revive him. However, when such an episode did occur, the hospital staff dramatically ignored the DNR order and proceeded to his resuscitation. They were favoring a sanctity-of-life perspective or else were protecting their staff and institution from unfavorable comment or possible litigation, or perhaps both. This was a high profile case! The hospital did not want any public criticism that suggested active euthanasia, which in 1988 was not as succinctly defined in professional circles, morally or legally, as it is today. In resuscitating the patient, the hospital staff, in my opinion, clearly violated the patient's rights and wishes as specified in his advance directive and as agreed upon by his physicians and his wife. It was a covenant recorded in his hospital medical chart. The family decided not to make an issue of that violation of the fiduciary relationship that existed between the patient and family on the one hand and the physician and hospital on the other. They rather chose to take the patient home under privately acquired medical supervision. I would argue that when one looks at the Schiavo case and all of the social and legal rancor that surrounded the case, this family seems to have made a very wise decision.

There is no civil or moral law that requires that a patient in this, or any other medical condition, be maintained in a hospital, unless there is evidence of physical abuse or criminal neglect at home. Reasonable persons and their surrogates may refuse efforts to be institutionalized, unless it appears that they are mentally incompetent. It is legal to be born at home; it is also legal to die at home. Ninety years ago, 75-80 percent of the persons who died in the United States did so at home. In third-world countries today, that percentage or greater still holds true. That figure has been dramatically reversed in the United States, so that now 75-80 percent in the United States die in a hospital, nursing facility, or institutional hospice. However, there appears to be a growing inclination, with the aid of home-health services and home hospice assistance, to reverse those figures somewhat.

John Doe II's wife, family, and physicians concluded, therefore, that his right to medical self-determination was being compromised, that he should be dismissed from the hospital and taken to the home of a family member, that the nutrition/hydration tube be withdrawn, and that he be lovingly cared for and palliated (pain and discomfort relief) until his imminent natural death. To do so would not be the underlying cause of his death. On the contrary, that end-stage process of finitude was set in motion by the arterial blockage, brain stem stroke, and subsequent mini strokes. In my opinion, transferring the patient from the hospital to a family home on May 16, 1988, was the right thing to do, if it were something that the family was able to manage. The advance directive that he executed some years earlier was honored. To have kept him in a horribly debilitated state for an indeterminable period of time in a hospital intensive care unit hooked up to machines with zero quality of life, simply because of the legal and moral indecisiveness of the period, would have been inhumane for the patient and the family. In addition, it honored the patient's advance directives, which is a consistent theme in this book.

Eight days later, on May 23, John Doe II died in the home of a family member, surrounded by his loved ones and his pastor. A home health-care nurse was secured to administer palliative care until the end. That care was monitored by their next-door physician friend and, when death came, another physician friend was present to sign the death certificate. That physician said to me retrospectively, "All of the family stakeholders were in agreement with the selected course of action." Both physicians, as well as those on the hospital medical staff, had earlier concluded that he would not get any better and was in a state worse than death. Near the end, he had zero quality of life. The scene at the family home was an accepting and peaceful one. If it had to happen, it was a "good death," which, we saw earlier, is the precise definition of the Greek word *eu-thanatos*, that is, *euthanasia*, passively rendered. He was afforded a natural death with significant dignity.

With a consistent medical indication of locked-in syndrome, at first able to participate in eye communication, John Doe II's mental response capability had diminished in the latter half of his hospital stay of almost four weeks. During the entire time, his wife was also concerned about their three-year-old daughter. A recorded message from "daddy's little girl" was brought to the hospital, but it was uncertain as to the patient's reaction. Desiring to be at her husband's bedside as much as possible, the wife and mother wanted to see to the emotional needs of their little girl as well. Realizing the dilemma, the family pediatrician telephoned and suggested that psychological assistance be sought for their daughter who suddenly had been separated from her father by his illness. Immediately the services of a child psychologist were secured and continued through the next year. It was that professional who guided them in having the three-year-old visit her dad before his death.

Years later, in discussing with me her own physically and spiritually draining experiences in the clinical netherworld, the patient's wife reflected on what she considered to be collateral damage to herself. During those emotionally charged weeks of her husband's sudden illness, death, and aftermath, there was so much to be done: anxious presence at the bedside, not knowing whether she was helping or hurting, immediate needs of her daughter at home, respectful concerns for other family members at all levels, the final searching moments, funeral arrangements, husband's law office to be cleared and closed, bills to be paid, estate and probate issues, persons to be thanked. There was a long list of necessary tasks, some more important and more immediately demanding than others.

Several times she commented on the fact that in doing so much, she had not seen to her own needs. The pastor of her church had transferred a short time before their family crisis. She felt alone and scared. The husband whom she loved was gone. She was a thirty-seven-year-old widow with a three-year-old daughter. "In a sense," she said, "my survival instinct kicked in."

Her emotional reaction was a natural phenomenon within a crisis experience. Faced with corresponding situations, many grieving persons have shared similar feelings and thoughts, and much has been written about the grief processes resulting from tragic events such as these. During the course of the bedside vigils, the long periods in the intensive care waiting rooms, and the public and private memorializing afterwards, scores of people come and go in addition to the professional health-care providers: family, friends, acquaintances, and many who knew your spouse, but whom you had not met before. Suddenly, it's over. As Kipling observed in his poem, life's important and crowded moments may suddenly become *Recessional*: "The captains and the kings depart." Others return to their schedules and seemingly predictable patterns of life. Then, there is just you—and a little girl! The patterns of your lives have suddenly and irrevocably changed. No wonder a person feels alone and fearful. The grief remains and unendingly tempers the future. Death, though a natural occurrence, must be recognized, understood, and dealt with by one's self, with the aid of family, friends, spiritual advisor, or often with the aid of a professional psychological counselor.

Jean-Dominique Bauby (The Butterfly)[3]

In the north of France, near Pas de Calais, there is a lovely village on the edge of still lovelier beaches, just across the channel from England. The renovated naval hospice/rehab hospital there at Berck-sur-Mur, formerly was a nineteenth-century medical facility for children recovering from long-term illnesses. It was there, in this picturesque but oft-times depressing clinical setting that one of France's high profile and most popular citizens awakened after several weeks in a coma—slowly to be made aware that he was almost completely paralyzed. From his nose downward, Jean-Dominique Bauby could not move, yet he could think, smell, and cry. As the mental stupor began to diminish, he was told by physicians that he was medically compromised by an anomaly called locked-in syndrome, resulting from a brain-stem stroke weeks earlier, on December 8, 1995. Cognitively active, he was able to communicate only by blinking his left eye in response to questions, once for yes and twice for no.

One has to be daunted with the suddenness by which such a medical calamity impacted the lives of Bauby and the two previous John Does near the mid-point of their potential ages and perhaps at the height of their careers. John Doe I was forty-seven, and John Doe II was fifty-one when they were afflicted. The Parisian "Jean-Do," as Jean-Dominique Bauby was affectionately called by his then-current lady friend Florence, was forty-three, the editor-in-chief of the very popular *Elle Magazine*. The publication, focusing on the interests and concerns of women, has offices in major cities worldwide. When hearing of the paralyzing condition in which the prestigious Bauby was "locked," many simply could not visualize it, since he was such an international symbol of vitality and achievement.

At the outset, Bauby was buoyed with hope shared by his physicians that new technologies and treatment might translate into measured improvement and significant recovery over time. Believing that his particular locked-in state was less severe than some others, Dominique Bauby accepted the challenge of a life with exceedingly poor quality and deprivation. He had good reasons to persevere. There were two children by a former spouse, eight-year-old daughter, Celeste, and ten-year-old son, Theophile, both of whom he adored. Still "mentally" alert and still the journalist, Bauby courageously sought to give the world a unique view of a person in this rare medical condition. Though physically locked-in, he made the decision to have some of his thoughts and experiences recorded in an amazing book, which he entitled *The Diving Bell and* the *Butterfly.* The portrayal of himself as one who is perpetually confined within an oppressive "diving chamber" sustained by compressed air is a graphic description of the paralysis impairing his bodily movement. At the same time, he pictured himself as a "butterfly" that soars beyond the physical imprisonment into the ethereal regions of creative thoughts and memories.

Transferring his recollections, contemplations, and rehab experiences is a story in itself—narratives shared by one who cannot move or talk—one who communicates only by the blinking of his eye. The effort was painstakingly accomplished with the aid of a young woman, Claude Mendebil. She interacted with Bauby in crafting an alphabetical scheme, used somewhat by others in similar medical situations. One by one, letters of the alphabet were spelled out by Claude, and when the desired letter was pronounced, Bauby blinked his eye affirmatively. Correspondingly, Claude recorded it and then meticulously moved to another after transferring the letter by pencil onto her notepad. In French, English, or most other languages, certain letters appear more frequently, so they were respectively placed at the beginning of the alphabetical list of letters to advance the process more rapidly and efficiently. With a brief prologue, followed by twenty-eight terse chapters, Bauby uniquely dictated a story of his journey through the dark uncertainties of the clinical netherworld and his mental efforts to escape to a higher level, if only temporarily: "Through the frayed curtain at my window, a wan glow announces the break of day. My heels hurt, my head weighs a ton, and something like a giant invisible diving bell holds my whole body prisoner. . . . Up until then, I had never even heard of the brain stem."[4]

Having begun his extraordinary literary gem weeks after waking from a coma in the naval hospital at Berck-Plage (beach), Jean-Dominique Bauby described his depressive encounters with patients not unlike himself. One other patient had experienced a vascular accident, similar but perceptually more severe than his own locked-in condition. There were aging patients seeking arduously to overcome strokes, while he observed young male and female athletes in differing levels of recovery from a variety of sports accidents leaving them with paraplegia and quadriplegia. But, focusing on the sad plight of others over a period slightly more than two years only made him ponder the grim state of himself.

Intermingled artistically with such sorrowful physical and visual encounters are pleasant memories of Bauby's former halcyon days when life was somewhat peaceful and calm: days and nights filled with friendship, art, music, romantic interludes, and testy but manageable professional demands. There is a mental and emotional flow back and forth in his love for and visits with his children, Celeste and Theophile, visits which at times left him in tears and contemplation over what their lives would become. To have orderly transferred his thoughts and treasured memories and edited them at the same time, was a remarkable demonstration of mental tenacity. The process itself revealed the personal knowledge of the arts and gifted attributes of an unusually talented man brought physically low by an untimely and devastating natural event.

The penultimate chapter describes the somewhat frantic moments of the brain-stem stroke occurring near the home where his children lived with their mother outside of Paris, along with the desperate automobile trip to the hospital at Mantes ten miles away. After two months in tandem with Claude during the summer following the December arterial accident, the book effort was complete, at least on his part. The final chapter closes with Bauby glumly aware of his own existential situation, speculating whether the collective data would translate into a book, and wondering if he would ever be freed from his oppressive prison. Over the next six months the book was prepared for publication, and on March 9, 1997, it was released to the public, two days before he died at Berck-Plage. He was forty-five years old.

Though diagnosed with the same medical anomaly, the respective rights to autonomy and to medical self-determination played out in three different ways for these three unfortunates, who were immanently beset with an incurable disease. I would submit that each of the three made an autonomous decision that was right for him. John Doe I, after returning to consciousness in the intensive unit of a Nashville medical center with the diagnosis of locked–in syndrome, was advised by his physicians that his condition was incurable. There was no reasonable chance of recovery. Life supports offered no clinical benefit other than to maintain the status quo—a state of abject medical futility. He had no previously executed advance directives, nor were they necessary. Though completely paralyzed, his mind was clear and he chose to have the life supports withdrawn, a recognition that, for him, life had descended to lowest ebb possible in a netherworld environment. It was his call, and the professional staff was supportive of his decision.

John Doe II, collapsed at home and subsequently stabilizing there, was taken to a Nashville medical center. Initial examination led to a diagnosis of transient ischemic attack, a mild and fleeting stroke, usually presenting no immediate danger. Kept over that night for observation and further tests, he sustained a subsequent stroke of the basilar artery in his midbrain and brain stem, which left him with locked-in syndrome. Initially, he could communicate with blinking eye responses to questions. Otherwise, he was totally paralyzed. Several days later, still in intensive care, his condition worsened to the point of unresponsiveness. There was no hope for improvement or recovery. Earlier conversation with family and friends, and written advance directives indicated preference for no "heroic measures," if, in fact, they were ever medically indicated. In the face of hospital reluctance to withdraw life supports after four weeks, the family took their loved one home and rendered medical palliative care only, satisfied that they had done the right thing—nature had already made its decision and the patient's advance directive only confirmed it. The family had no desire to make a public display of this tragic situation and avoided a court contest that they believed would serve absolutely no useful purpose.

The "Butterfly," John-Dominique Bauby, in turn, was given initial hope by the physicians at Berck that his locked-in situation might possibly improve with treatment and perhaps lead to a reasonable recovery. Willfully subjecting himself to physically discomforting life-support systems and laboriously committed to the creation of a small but unique book detailing his oppressed existence, Bauby set about to show his friends and the world that he was more than a vegetable. Despite his fortitude, within fifteen months he was dead from the natural cerebral accident, but not before his book had been published and released. There is currently a film about Bauby, having been staged and filmed in Hollywood.

    The individual right to medical self-determination, codified in law, therefore continues here and throughout the netherworld journey, as a primary factor in the decision-making process. It blends the right of the patient or surrogate to be informed, along with the right of consent or refusal of treatment. Each of the three locked-in patients made autonomous decisions, and each did what was right for him. Though there were similarities in these three cases of locked-in syndrome, they were not the same. No two medical cases ever are!

Chapter XIII

Amyotrophic Lateral Sclerosis

Lou Gehrig[1]

In 1925 first baseman Lou Gehrig joined Babe Ruth in the starting lineup of the Yankees. What a magnificent career followed! Lou Gehrig accomplished 13 consecutive seasons of 100 or more runs batted in. He played with the Yankees in 7 World Series (34 World Series games averaging .361, with 10 home runs and 31 runs batted in). During his 17-year career with the Yankees, Gehrig hit a total of 493 home runs, tied an all-time record of four homers in one game, and had a lifetime batting average of .340. Lou won the Triple Crown in 1934, with a batting average of 365 combined with 49 home runs and an amazing 165 runs batted in![2]

It should have been the height of his career, but in the latter part of the 1938 season and the early part of the 1939 season, almost everyone associated with major league baseball had observed that something dramatic was affecting the capacity of Lou to perform well in the game that he loved so much. His manager and coaches, his fellow team-mates, the umpires, the opposition, the fans, the sportswriters—and most importantly, Lou, himself, found it inexplicable!

As team captain, Lou Gehrig eventually took himself out of the New York starting lineup on May 2, 1939.[3] Up to that point, "Iron Man" Lou had participated in 2,130 consecutive games; a record finally surpassed 59 years later by Cal Ripkin, Jr., playing for the Baltimore Orioles in 1998. Experiencing unexplainable loss of physical dexterity, Gehrig benched himself for what he personally described as "the good of the game."' Not knowing the reason for the dramatic slump, Lou was even then making a sure but certain descent into his personal netherworld. Unable to play baseball was bad enough; it became more foreboding than that! He died twenty-five months later, on June 2, 1941, of an illness called amyotrophic lateral sclerosis, which now bears his name, "Lou Gehrig's disease." He was thirty-eight years of age.

The final stages of Lou Gehrig's disease (ALS) are ultimately symptomatic of those clinical characteristics exhibited by locked-in syndrome, considered in the previous chapter. Locked-in syndrome occurs abruptly, concisely, shutting down the entire body's vegetative action except for the upper brain (cognitive) functions. If one survives the initial trauma, the mentally aware person is trapped within a paralyzed and dysfunctional body, requiring a total mechanical life-support system for an interim period. With no known cure, ordinarily it leads to death within a relatively short period of time.

The symptoms of Lou Gehrig's disease, on the other hand, begin slowly, almost tantalizingly, to become manifest in very subtle ways: the initial fumbling with the most elementary items such as the use of eating utensils or picking up a bat, slight twitching of arm or shoulder muscles, the incapacity of lifting the feet, with subsequent shuffling gait. With time, the symptoms exacerbate until the body arrives at total muscular and nervous system failure and, resembling locked-in syndrome, ultimately requires respirators, feeding tubes, and other medical regimen. The end results of both diseases, locked-in syndrome and ALS, are dramatically similar. A definitive description of the medical anomaly and its impact on the human body is offered by The National Institute of Neurological Disorders and Stroke:

> Amyotrophic lateral sclerosis (ALS), sometimes called Lou Gehrig's disease, is a rapidly progressive, invariably fatal neurological disease that attacks the nerve cells (neurons) responsible for controlling voluntary muscles. In ALS, both the upper motor neurons and the lower motor neurons degenerate or die, ceasing to send messages to muscles. Unable to function, the muscles gradually weaken, waste away, and twitch. Eventually the ability of the brain to start and control voluntary movement is lost. Individuals with ALS lose their strength and ability to move their arms, legs, and body. When muscles in the diaphragm and chest wall fail, individuals lose the ability to

breathe without ventilatory support. In most cases the disease does not impair a person's mind, personality, intelligence or memory, nor does it affect a person's ability to see, smell, taste, hear or recognize touch....
No cure has been found for ALS.

There is currently only one drug that has shown to have any effect on Lou Gehrig's Disease, according to the Neurological National Institute. "Riluzole," they report, "is believed to reduce damage to motor neurons and may prolong survival by several months, mainly in those with difficulty in swallowing."

So, the time arrives when the patient and physician must decide if the medical treatments and life supports will continue and under what set of excruciating circumstances. Lou Gehrig was offered no such choice. His death from amyotrophic lateral sclerosis in 1941 occurred in the recesses of a New York Hospital without the aid of antibiotics, respirators, and feeding tubes, all of which later became treatments of choice in withholding and withdrawing for patients suffering from ALS and locked–in syndrome. As compared with medical intensive care units of today, those in 1941 were not far removed from those of the nineteenth century. Still offering no cure, medical science with its respirators, feeding tubes, and antibiotics, has extended the time line, creating awesome quality of life issues and financial burdens preceding inevitable death. Lou Gehrig lived barely two years after his diagnosis of ALS in 1939. Most victims today live for three to five years following diagnosis, and ten percent survive three times longer than the average.

In 1984, I first became involved in clinical ethics. At that time, many physicians, nurses, and other professionals opined and practiced that it was permissible to withhold treatment but not to withdraw it. As recently as 1998, the authors of the book *Clinical Ethics* observed, "One still hears in clinical settings such remarks as 'withholding treatment might be acceptable, but once it's started, we cannot withdraw,' or, 'would extubation be active or passive.' "[4] After life support was implemented, those treatments ordinarily had to remain in place until the patient died. Such was the morally flawed perspective of some clinicians and many in the lay public.

For those concerned about active euthanasia, suicide, and assisted suicide, this connection was often made. At the time there were numbers of physicians, nurses, philosophers, clergy, and clinical ethicists, including myself, along with some laypersons, who disagreed with such views. The terminology "proportionate care" appears to be more acceptable to many clinicians: such as the ones who authored *Clinical Ethics*. "This principle," they wrote, "states that a medical treatment is ethically mandatory to the extent that it is likely to confer greater benefit over its attendant burdens."[5]

Thus, we believe along with autonomy, the right to accept or refuse treatment, medical procedures that are non-beneficial to the patient can legally and morally be withheld or withdrawn. As if to test that kind of ethical and legal reasoning, two ALS cases surfaced almost simultaneously in the Nashville area in 1980s and were transitioned from hospital cases to court cases. Apparently, they were the first right-to-die cases to be litigated in Tennessee. In other parts of the country in the same period, similar episodes were occurring.

Jane Doe[6]

On the afternoon of February 5, 1990, a headline in the *Nashville Banner* read: "Woman sues for the right to die." The woman was identified only as "Jane Doe." Two months later, the second patient, Nancy Gamble, petitioned the court for relief from her respirator and for the right to negotiate or allow a natural death. The same lawyer, Mary Martin Schaffner, represented both medically compromised clients in the ensuing legal procedures in separate chancery courts and thus argued the cases in front of two different judges. Reports indicated that Attorney Schaffner represented these plaintiffs "pro bono," i.e., she accepted no fees for involvement in these important, time-consuming, and initial right-to-die cases in Tennessee.

Jane Doe, was a sixty-two-year-old woman who was initially diagnosed with Lou Gehrig's disease in 1982. She and her husband were the parents of several sons, and they lived in a rural area outside of Nashville. Gradually losing dexterity in her fingers and the capacity to grasp with her hands, she began to shuffle her feet as she walked. Series of tests under the scrutiny of her family physician, Nashville internist Dr. James Wilson, led to the conclusion that she was in the early stages of amyotrophic lateral sclerosis. Two years later, in early 1984, her condition worsened, and she was admitted to a Nashville hospital with a serious lung infection. Jane Doe was placed on a respirator to assist with her breathing, a technology that went home with her after several weeks and remained in place until her death in 1990. "She is locked in her body," Wilson said. "She deserves the right not to persist in a vegetative state, locked on a respirator, unable to communicate with her environment."[7]

Jane Doe, during her last six years, was bedridden and could not walk, talk, or feed herself. In addition to a feeding tube in her stomach, she could, with assistance, minimally swallow some fluids and very light food. That capacity, however, diminished as her illness progressed. Her method of communication was aided by a unique computer. In the latter stages of the disease, the computer was operated by the only finger that she could move, her right thumb. It was reported in local hospital ethics forums by Dr. Wilson that, after suffering with ALS for eight years, six of them on the respirator, Jane Doe struggled to type a three-word message, one letter at a time, onto her computer: "Set date die."[8]

Both patient and physician felt that it was ethically appropriate to make such a request and to facilitate it. But, considering the legal uncertainty of the time, they consulted with Attorney Schaffner, who advised them to seek a judgment in court to allow Dr. Wilson to do for Jane Doe what she could not physically do for herself, that is, to remove the respirator. "Certainly there is a need for a decision to be made in this situation because she is not able to exercise her right to die naturally," explained the lawyer to *Nashville Banner* newspaper reporter Bill Snyder and to the court in a brief.[9]

The Tennessee Right to Natural Death Act was legislated earlier in 1985 to give competent persons the right to execute a living will, which would become effective later, at the end of life, if they became incompetent. Patients can decide in advance, states the law, "as circumstances permit and to accept, refuse, withdraw from, or otherwise control decisions relating to the rendering of his or her own medical care." The strange twist in this case, however, is that Jane Doe was still competent to make her own decisions, while the law on living wills was written to become effective with incompetency. I would argue, therefore, that in filing her brief in the Chancery Court of C. Allen High, Attorney Mary Martin Schaffner spoke succinctly to the issue:

> Plaintiff submits that the right to direct her medical care when <u>competent</u> can be no less than her right to direct her care should she subsequently become <u>incompetent</u>—that is, plaintiff now has the right to direct her physician to withdraw the respirator that is artificially prolonging her life without exposing him to criminal or civil liability.[10]

So, Dr. Wilson was taken into Chancery Court by Jane Doe and her attorney, Mary Martin Schaffner, in this "friendly" lawsuit. They were not seeking reimbursement for damages but rather seeking a legal judgment on the right to have her life support systems removed, without the incrimination of assisted suicide or murder on the part of the compassionate physician. In his ruling the judge affirmed: "The law recognizes the existence of the right of a competent adult to make a voluntary and informed decision not to continue life-prolonging medical procedures."[11] A subsequent editorial in the *Nashville Banner* told the rest of the story—most of which appears here:

> Chancellor C. Allen High made a difficult decision Monday in ruling that a dying woman known only as Jane Doe has the right to have the respirator—the only thing keeping her alive—disconnected. This is believed to be Tennessee's first so-called right to die case. It doesn't set a legal precedent. But it does break new ground in a complex area of law and medicine that is being pushed to the fore by advances in medical technology and longer life spans. Some believe she shouldn't have that right—that by allowing the respirator to be turned off, society makes it easier to support suicides by disabled or terminally ill persons later. . . . Chancellor High even took the unusual step of holding court at Jane Doe's bedside, waiting patiently as she assured him through thumb signals that she realized the consequences of what she was asking and that the request was her true wish. That was a compassionate gesture that emphasized his determination to weigh the request carefully.[12]

Chancellor High's unique court process on this end-of-life case took place in the tranquil confines of a family dwelling in a rural area, the location of which was not revealed to the public. The removal of the life-support systems by Dr. Wilson followed several weeks later in the same setting. Though Jane Doe's nervous system had deteriorated to a point where almost all her bodily functions had shut down, she nevertheless had a clear mind and decision-making capacity. Autonomy, her right to determine her own destiny, one that did not impinge on the rights of anyone else, was a choice for her to make. She had a right, as has already been concluded in the preceding cases, to refuse treatment or, if initially accepted, to have it withdrawn later.

In neither case would withholding or withdrawing be tantamount to suicide, nor would it be it be a criminal act for Dr. Wilson to accede to her request for assistance at either level. Wilson earlier made that point very clear in an interview with *Nashville Banner* Senior Medical Writer Bill Snyder, "She is not asking for the right to commit suicide," he said, "because respirators are considered 'extraordinary means' of prolonging life." Then he added, "I think that represents termination of life due to a terminal disease."[13] Such medical principle was legally confirmed in Chancellor High's opinion. The physician, Dr. Wilson, was able to treat her with medicine, respirator, nutrition, and hydration in the first place only because she had given him permission to do so. It was her decision in consult with her physician, and not that of anyone else, to use medicine and technology to sustain her for a period near the end of life, and it was her decision to request of her physician that life supports be withdrawn. She had decided that it was time for her to die, since life for her was an existence of almost zero quality. Jane Doe's death was encompassed with dignity—it was facilitated within the privacy of her own home, thus not abrogating any institutional policies or procedures—and it was peaceful—it was moral—and it was deemed by the court to be legal. Her death was her own to claim.

Nancy Gamble[14]

The second legal request in Metropolitan Nashville for a patient's right to die occurred in relatively frenetic contrast to the first one. Nancy Gamble also was afflicted with Lou Gehrig's disease. At the time of her lawsuit, she had been a patient at Nashville Baptist Hospital. In the debilitating stages of the disease she was placed on a respirator and feeding tube. Her final fourteen months of life, with the exception of two trips to nursing facilities, were spent on life supports in a hospital within the bustle of mid-town Nashville. She was moved to a nursing home in August 1989 but returned to Baptist Hospital twice after that. By early December, Gamble was no longer able to leave the hospital. One of her physicians, Neurologist Michael J. Kaminski, who examined her on March 16, 1990, said in an affidavit filed later with the court:

> Nancy Gamble is now in the terminal stages of ALS. She cannot walk, talk, feed herself or breathe on her own. She can communicate only by mouthing words or shaking her head . . . the patient is aware she will die within minutes after the ventilator is removed. . . . She mouthed the words 'I want to die.'[15]

After Gamble began to negotiate with her physician on her wishes to have the life supports withdrawn, she and her internist, Dr. James Sullivan, were personally vexed by the hospital's reticence to consider it. In turn they sought attorney Mary Martin Schaffner for legal advice and assistance. The woman was on Medicaid and the attorney was representing her pro bono, without charge. Nancy Gamble, age 50, was unmarried; she had no children, but there was a sister, who, according to her attorney "fully supports her decision."[16] In a separate affidavit, Nashville psychiatrist William Kenner who had examined Gamble several days earlier said he believed she has made the decision on her own and has not been "coerced by others."[17] When a lawsuit was filed in the Metro Nashville Chancery Court of Robert Brandt, the word spread to the news media (through United Press International as far away as the *Los Angeles Times*) and to a variety of citizen groups, including one with the acronym ADAPT. This latter group, Americans Disabled for Attendant Programs Today, also filed briefs with the court seeking to prevent the respirator removal. In the legal brief relative to Gamble, they expressed anxiety about "further movement down the slippery slope to euthanasia of individuals whom society may perceive as unwanted burdens."[18]

Earlier the group had followed the proceedings of the Jane Doe case. As indicated in the newspaper editorial relative to Chancellor High's Jane Doe decision, they saw both of these cases as threats to disabled persons such as themselves living with severe disabilities. Suicide and assisted suicide implications in my opinion were wrongly ascribed by ADAPT to all patients with terminal illness who might request that their life supports be removed. In the legal filing they claimed that Gamble was being denied "the same qualified crisis intervention and suicide prevention services that would be provided to anyone else."[19] However, Attorney Schaffner had already given assurance to the court that Gamble was mentally alert and regularly engaged in consultations with a psychiatrist and neurologist along with her repeated requests for removal of her respirator.[20] The decision of the court affirmed that requests for the removal of life supports were legally and morally valid requests, and in no way were suicidal in nature.

Additional concern, however, was expressed by ADAPT and others in public demonstrations at the courthouse and in the lobby of the Nashville hospital. "Terminal illness should not be used," they said, "to justify a wholesale abandonment of society's policies designed to protect human life."[21] I would argue that ADAPT, ironically, was attempting to deny the right of privacy and self-determination for patients like Nancy Gamble, meanwhile claiming for themselves the right to be left alone and the right to choose their own quality of life within their disabilities. The final judgment of Chancellor Robert Brandt, in the Nancy Gamble request for a natural death, appears to concur with such an argument, as did the judgment of Chancellor High in the Jane Doe Case:

> This action was heard on April 10, 1990. After considering the evidence, the court is of the opinion that a mentally competent adult who is fully informed of his/her prognosis, the medical alternatives, and the risk of withdrawing medical treatment may decide to refuse treatment if the patient's chart contains typed, signed statements from two independent physicians that the patient is competent and fully informed of the consequences of refusing treatment. If these criteria are met, court authorization is not required unless

there are conflicting opinions between doctors and/or family members of the patient. Further, if these criteria are met no civil or criminal liability will attach to health care providers who may participate in or allow withdrawal of medical treatment.[22]

On April 11, 1990, a headline in the *Nashville Banner*, Section B, appeared in bold print: **"Woman dies quietly after winning case."** Nancy Gamble had sued Nashville Baptist Hospital for the right to die. The article went on to state, "A Nashville woman . . . had her respirator disconnected about 8 a.m. today . . . [and] died peacefully about 15 minutes later, her attorney said."[23] Nancy Gamble's sister, her physician James Sullivan M.D., and Gamble's favorite nurse, along with Attorney Schaffner, were at the hospital during the process but were not present in the room, according to a report in the *Nashville Banner* the next day.[24] Five years earlier, the State Senate in 1985, by a vote of 25-5, had passed the Tennessee Right to Natural Death Act. With these two successfully adjudicated cases, the right to health-care self determination was significantly enhanced.

One issue should be in perspective now. We have not discussed in this book the moral and legal ramifications of suicide or assisted suicide. Such debate must be undertaken by someone else, or if by this ethicist, in a separate well-defined format. The discussion here, acknowledging neocortical death (PVS) and impending death (locked-in syndrome and ALS), along with a concurrent right to have treatment withheld and withdrawn, merits greater clarification among the rank and file members of our contemporary society. That is what we have tried to do in *So Falls a Sparrow*.

Karen Ann Quinlan, Paul Brophy, Nancy Cruzan, and Terri Schiavo sustained irreversible non-traumatic but catastrophic insults to their brain. In each case it was morally and legally argued that none of these would have wished to remain in such a debilitated state. Not one of these was any longer a sentient person, and medical supports were belatedly withdrawn and justice finally prevailed, but only after judicial decisions were rendered in the courts in petitions submitted by their surrogates. Hopefully, such cases have served as moral and legal precedence for many who have followed in their train.

As already noted, there is no cure for locked-in syndrome or for ALS. Thus, clear-minded physically locked-in patients make the call, usually very early along a spectrum of tragic futility. Ordinarily, the decision to withdraw comes swiftly. On the other hand, with ALS patients the wasting away of the body proceeds comparatively slow but decidedly complete and, near the end, is not unlike the tragic consequences of locked-in syndrome. Professor Maguire reasons, "In sum, then, death has lost its medical and moral simplicity. We know it now as a process, not a moment, and we have the means to extend or shorten the process."[25]

It is my view, along with a consensus of others mentioned, that ordinary refusal of non-beneficial medical treatment by a mentally competent terminally ill patient through verbal or written advanced directives, or through one's health-care surrogate, is not deemed to be suicide. Nor is it assisted suicide or murder when a physician accedes to the request of a patient or surrogate that non-beneficial life supports be withdrawn, an inordinately moral request considering the multiple crises often at hand.

Medical and religious enthusiasts, joined by the purists in the sanctity-of-life perspective, indeed are to be commended for their tenacious advocacy of the value and sacredness of human life. This author joins them in upholding those principles. But they cannot argue for its infinity or ignore valid claims of futility or zero quality of life pitted against its sanctity. The finitude of life, thus, has a quintessential place in the end-of-life dialogue. Biological life, as we know and experience it on planet Earth, has its bounds and limitations. Regardless of the rationale for our cultural penchant for denial, the technological captivity of patients in the clinical netherworld at the end of life leads to enormous emotional and financial burdens being placed on patients, families, and the health-care system of this country and is a profound justice issue.

Epilogue

So falls a sparrow to the ground—a continuing phenomenon in one form or another since life first emerged many ages ago in the primeval seas and virgin forests of planet Earth. The eighth-century BC Hebrew psalmist affirms, "Even the sparrow finds a home and the swallow a nest for herself . . . her young."[1] And, Jesus of Nazareth taught reassuringly, "Are not two sparrows sold for a penny? Yet not one of them will fall to the ground apart from your Father."[2] Even with God's notice, the sparrow still falls. For most Judeo-Christians, each nesting and each fall are part of a broadly-based, purposely driven theological spectrum. For secular naturalists, they are part of an all-encompassing biological determinism of birth, death, and rebirth on planet Earth. For many others of us, who believe that we do not live in a value-free universe, they are an abridgement of both perspectives. The conclusions of physician Sherwin Nuland are appropriate here:

> Nature has a job to do. It does its job by the method that seems most suited to each individual who its powers have created. It has made this one susceptible to heart disease and that one to stroke and yet another to cancer, some after a long time on this earth and some after a time much too brief at least by our own reckoning. The animal economy has formed the circumstances by which each generation is to be succeeded by the next. Against the relentless forces and cycles of nature there can be no lasting victory.[3]

Though the ingenious and spirited human species has been the dominant presence in nature's ongoing life-and-death cycle, it too, like the sparrow, returns to the earth's dust—yet, persons of faith believe that there is hope for perpetuity beyond this life. Gazing upon the persons gathered around him, Jesus reassured them, "So do not be afraid; you are of more value than many sparrows."[4] Infinite sacredness and evolutionary value are in each person's life and in each person's death. The everlasting drama is not without purpose and ongoing meaning.

Appendix

A. Acknowledgments

Gratitude is extended to the following who, respectively, have been involved in the author's personal journey through the fields of political, social, and medical ethics.

Professors: Bill Barnes, Don Beisswenger, Howard L. Harrod, Thomas Ogletree, Peter Paris, Holmes Rolston, Andy Watts.

Attorneys: Lee Barfield, Alan Yuspeh, Attorney/Professor David Smith.

Hospital CEOs: Ed Stainback, Bill Gracey, Bryan Deering, Robert Klein, and Jeff Whitehorn.

Clinical Ethicist: Ron Huff.

Deans: John Chapman, Louis J. Bernard.

Physicians: William P. Dutton, Eric Raefsky, Jay Jacobson, Norman Sims, Hayden Lambert, Ken Iserson, Thomas Frist, Sr., James T. Robertson, Carl Gessler, Luther Smith, Stephen Pont.

Medical Chancellors: Roscoe Robinson, Eugene Fowinkle.

Summit Chief Nursing Officers: Cathy Gracey, Mary Ann Angle.

Registered Nurses: Jackie Price, Amanda Stephens, Beth Davidson.

Hospital Pharmacist: Jack Cronk.

Donelson Hospital Board of Trustees member: Willie McDonald.

Judicial Chancellor: Carol McCoy.

Special thanks to families and friends related to cases: A. J. and Shirley Coleman, John Scoble, Raymond White, Joan Warvel Mullins, Peggy and Bill White, and The Rev. Dr. Robert N. Watkin. *A host of case manager nurses and social workers* at Donelson, Summit, and Skyline Medical Centers.

Special thanks, also, are extended to copy editor Nancy Provost, and also to Freda Dye, grandsons Luke Johnson and Caleb Johnson, and son Dennis Crumby for computer technical assistance; a special appreciation to Jody Johnson for textual emendations and to Donna Pritchett for detailing the images of the brain. Grandson and Univ. of Kentucky Law student Luke Johnson is deserving of my deep appreciation for textual emendations and for steering the publication process through Creatspace (hard copy) and Kindle Direct Publishing (electronic edition).

B. Notes

All references cited in the Great Books of the Western World series will fall under the format exhibited in reference no.8 of Chapter 1, and will thereafter appear under the limited rubric: title. volume, Great Books, and page number, along with author's name when necessary for identification. The same rubric will apply to citations in *The Great Ideas Today* publications, as appearing in reference no. 18 in chapter 1.

Part One
1. William Osler, "Quotes," Osler Society of New York, http://oslersociety.org/index.php/by-osler (2010).

Chapter I
1. John S. Mackenzie, *A Manual of Ethics* (New York: W. B. Cline, 1897; Hinds, Noble, and Eldridge, 1901), 1.
2. Daniel C. Maguire, *Ethics: A Complete Method for Moral Choice* (Minneapolis: Fortress Press, 2010), 30.
3. Eric J. Cassell, *The Healer's Art*: *A New Approach to the Doctor Patient Relationship*, (Philadelphia: J.B. Lippincott, 1976), 87.
4. Edmund. D. Pelligrino, *Humanism and the Physician* (Knoxville: University of Tennessee Press, 1979), 17.
5. Second Samuel 23:1, KJV.
6. Psalm 8:1, 3-6. NRSV.
7. Robert A. Veatch, *A Theory of Medical Ethics* (New York: Basic Books, 1981), 29-30.
8. *Hippocratic Writings*, trans., Francis Adams, vol. 10, The Great Books (Chicago: Encyclopedia Britannica, 1952), ix.
9. Ibid.
10. Pelligrino, *Humanism*, 97-98.
11. *Hippocratic Writings*, xiii.
12. Hazel J. Markwell and Barry, F. Brown, "Bioethics for Clinicians: 27," Catholic Bioethics *Canadian Medical Association Journal* (July 24, 2001): 165(2).
13. Karl Barth, *Church Dogmatics*, *III/4*, *The Doctrine of Creation*, ed. G.W. Bromiley and T.F. Torrance, trans. A.T. Mackay, T.H.L. Parker, Harold Knight, Henry Kennedy, John Marks, (Edinburgh: T & F Clark, 1961), 324.

14. Ibid., 340.
15. Ibid., 341.
16. Council on Theology and Culture, "The Nature and Value of Human Life," *Minutes of the 121st General Assembly, Presbyterian Church in the United States* (Part One, Journal with Directory and Appendix) 1981, 288.
17. Thomas Jefferson, *American State Papers: The Declaration of Independence*, vol.43, Great Books, 1-3.
18. "Magna Carta, 1215 A.D." *The Making of the Bill of Rights*, part 4, arranged by George Anastuplo, The Great Ideas Today, ed. Mortimer J. Adler (Chicago: Encyclopaedia Britannica, 1991), 332.
19. Immanuel Kant, *The Critique of Pure Reason, The Critique Practical Reason, and Other Ethical Treatises, The Critique of Judgment* "General Introduction to the Metaphysic of Morals," vol.42, Great Books, 393.
20. Allen D. Verhey, "Luther's Freedom of a Christian and a Patient's Autonomy," *Bioethics and the Future of Medicine, A Christian Appraisal*, ed. John F. Kilner, Nigel M. de s. Cameron, and David Schiederrmayer (Grand Rapids: William B. Eeedman's, 1995), 81.
21. Ibid. 83.
22. Amos 5:11, 5:24, NRSV.
23. Micah 6:8, NRSV.
24. P.V.N. Myers, *A Short History of Ancient Times,* (Boston: Ginn and Company, 1889, 1906), 130.
25. Ibid., 129.
26. Ibid., 130.
27. Pelligrino, *Humanism*, 3.
28. Ibid., 95.
29. John McKenzie, *A Manuel of Ethics*, (New York: Hinds, Noble, and Eldridge, 1897), 14.
30. Kant., *Critique*, 377.
31. Marguerite Wilkerson, "Guilty," *Masterpieces of Religious Verse*, ed. James Delton Morrison (New York: Harper and Brothers, 1948), poem 1385, 421.31.
32. William Henry Roberts, *The Problem of Choice: An Introduction to Ethics*, quotes ethicist R.M. MacIver, (Boston: Ginn and Company, 1941), 211.

33. *Aristotle II*, vol. 9, book 3, Great Books, 358.
34. Ibid.
35. Richard M. Zaner, *Ethics and the Clinical Encounter*, (Englewood Cliffs, N. J.: Prentice Hall, 1988), 27.
36., Edmund Pelligrino, "The Virtuous Physician and the Ethics of Medicine," *Contemporary Issues in Bioethics*, ed. Tom L. Beauchamp and Le Roy Walters (Beverly, Mass.: Wadsworth Publishing, 1999), 46-52.
37. Zaner, *Ethics and the Clinical Encounter*.
38. Ibid., 319.

Chapter II
1. Summit Medical Center, Nashville, Tenn., Cardiac Care Rehab Unit.
2. Holmes Rolston, III, *Genes, Genesis, God* (Edinburgh: Cambridge Univ. Press, 1999), ix-x.
3. Ibid, 306.
4. Helen Keller, *My Religion* (New York; Doubleday Page, 1927; reissued in 1997 under the title *Light in My Darkness*).
5. Diane Schurr, *Time Magazine*, US Edition, June 14, 1999, Vol.153, No.123, (Online) Time 100.
6. Keller, *My Religion*, 142.
7. Rolston, *Genes*, 306.
8. Peggy White, mother of Mary Moore, shared Mary's story with this author, and all relevant data are used with her permission. Peggy and her husband, Bill White, live in Chattanooga.
9. National Institute of Neurological Disorders and Stroke. (Online) Free use of material when credit is given.
10. White, personal notes.
11. White, personal notes.
12. Harry E. Fosdick, *The Meaning of Prayer*, (New York: Associated Press, 1951), 2-3.
13. Satguru Sivaya, *Dancing with Siva*, "Scriptures Speak on Liberation" (India-USA: Himalyan Academy, 1997), 116.
14. "Buddhism," Wikipedia, sec.3.4 "Meditation," http://en.wikipedia.org/wiki/Bhuddism#Meditation.
15. "Salat: Muslim Prayer," Religion Facts, 08/08/06. "Salat is executed each day, at dawn, midday, afternoon, sunset, and evening." (Online), Published 03/17/04, updated.

16. Isaiah 40: 31, NRSV.
17. Matthew 6: 5-14, NRSV.
18. 2 Corinthians 4: 8-9a, NRSV.
19. I Thessalonians 5:17, NRSV
20. Unless otherwise indicated, biographical materials related to the life of Lorene White were shared with this author by her husband, Raymond White, and are used with his permission.
21. Mayo Clinic Staff, "Patent ductus arteriosus (PDA)," "Definition," MayoClinic.com. 1998-2011, http://www.mayoclinic.com/health/patent-ductus-arteriosus/DS00631.
22. Eisenmenger's Syndrome is named after Paul Wood Eisenmenger who first described the condition in 1897; Wikipedia, http://en.wikipedia.org/wiki/Eisenmenger%27s_syndrome.
23. William Aylott Orton, *The Liberal Tradition, A Study of the Social and Spiritual Conditions of Freedom* (New Haven: Yale University Press, 1945), 29.

Chapter III
1. Jon Russell, "Editorial," *Journal of Musculoskeletal Pain* 8, no.3 (2000).
2. John F. Peppin, "Physician Values and Neutrality," *Bioethics and the Future of Medicine: A Christian Appraisal*, ed. John F. Kilner, Nigel M. de S. Cameron, and David Schiedemayer (Grand Rapids, Mich., and London: Eerdmans and Paternoster Press, 1995), 37.
3. American Medical Association, "Code of Medical Ethics: Current Opinions with Annotations," (American Medical Association, 2004), 2.035-2.037.
4. Stratton Hill, "When Will Adequate Pain Treatment Be the Norm?" *JAMA* 274, no. 23 (December 20, 1995), Editorials 1881.
5. Symposium on Pain Management Aimed at Medical School Students (New Haven, Conn.: Yale University Office of Public Affairs, May, 16, 2008), http://opac.yale.edu/news/article.aspx?id=5840.
6. I. Pilowski, *Curriculum on Pain for Medical Schools*, (International Association for the Study of Pain, 2011). http://www.iap-pain.org/AM/Template.cfm?Section=Home&Template=CM/

HTMLDisplay.cf.m&contentID=1807.
7. Eric Raefsky, M.D., Oncologist, Summit Medical Center, Nashville, Tenn., memo written April 14, 1992.
8. Bruce D. White, D.O., J.D., Director of Alden March Bioethics Institute and Professor of Pediatrics, Albany Medical College, Board Certified Pediatrician, Pharmacist and an Attorney with fellowship training in Clinical Medical Ethics.
9. Claudia Dreifus, "A Conversation with Robert Martenson" *New York Times*, sec. D2, January 20, 2009.
10. Ibid.
11. The story of Ruth Stanley was experienced by this author in his role of pastor to Ruth's daughter, Joan, some of it at the bedside of the patient, along with other data shared by Joan. Used with permission by family.
12. Paul Ramsey, *The Patient as Patient: Explorations in Medical Ethics* (New Haven and London: Yale University Press, 1970), 133.

Chapter IV
1. John Naisbett, *Megatrends: Ten New Directions Transforming our Lives,* (New York: Warner Books, 1982, 1984), 51.
2. Daniel Maguire, *The Moral Revolution: A Christian Humanist Vision,* (San Francisco: Harper and Row, 1986), 238.
3. Fosdick, *Meaning of Prayer*, entire book.
4. Fosdick, *Meaning of Prayer*, 120.
5. Patient Self-Determination Act, passed in 1990 by US Congress as an amendment to the Budget Reconciliation Act, became effective December 1, 1991. Wikipedia, http://en.wikipedia.org/wiki/Patient_Self-Determination_Act.
6. See Cruzan Case, ch. 10 within manuscript or online, Cruzan vs. Director of Missouri Dept. of Health, June 25, 1990. Decided in favor of withholding/withdrawing care, but upheld Missouri in its requirement of clear and convincing evidence as to patient's wishes.
7. National Conference of Catholic Bishops, "Ethical and Religious Directives for Catholic Health Care Services," (Washington, D.C.: United States Catholic Conference, 1995), part 5, article 57, 22-23.

8. "Life Abundant: Values, Choices and Health Care, The Responsibility and Role of the Presbyterian Church, U.S.A," Policy Statement adopted by the 200th. General Assembly, PCUSA (Louisville: Office of the General Assembly, 1988), 4.
9. Sherwin B. Nuland, *How We Die: Reflections on Life's Final Chapter.* (New York: Vintage Books, 1995), 264.
10, Margaret Pabst Battin, Quote of Seneca, *Ending Life: Ethics and the Way We Die* (New York: Oxford University Press, 2005), 5.
11. Nuland, *How We Die*, 265.

Chapter V
1. Thoughts shared in a personal evaluation by Holmes Rolston, Ph. D., University Distinguished Professor of Philosophy at Colorado State University. He is best known for his publications and contributions to environmental ethics, science, and religion, and is considered to be the "Father of environmental ethics." In 1997-98 he delivered the Gifford Lectures at the University of Edinburgh on the subject "Genes, Genesis, and God," which were published by Cambridge Press in 1999. In 2003 he was awarded the prestigious Templeton Prize in Religion, an annual award presented by the Templeton Foundation to a person who, in the estimation of the judges, "has made an exceptional contribution to affirming life's spiritual dimension, whether through insight, discovery, or practical works."
2. Psalm 90:10, KJV.
3. Matthew 10:29, KJV.
4. Holmes Rolston, *Science and Religion: A Critical Survey* (New York: Random House, 1987), 135-36.
5. Jonathan Swift, "Thoughts on Religion," vol. 1, chapter 15, *Writings on Religion and the Church*, The Literature Network, http://www.online-literature.com/view.php/religion-church-vol-one/15?term=.
6. Ernest Becker, *The Denial of Death,* (New York: The Free Press, A Division of Macmillan Publishing, 1973), ix.
7. Ibid, 2.
8. Miska Miles, *Annie and the Old One* (New York: Little, Brown Young Readers, May 30, 1985).

9. John Muir, *A Thousand Mile Walk to the Gulf*, (New York: Houghton Mifflin, 1916, renewed 1944 by Ellen Muir Funk), 70-71.
10. Will Durant, *Story of Civilization: Part I, Our Oriental Heritage* (New York: Simon and Schuster, 1954), 148-49.
11. Jessica Mitford, *The American Way of Death*, (New York: Simon and Schuster, 1963), 16.
12. John S. De Mott, "The High Cost of Dying," AARP Bulletin, 50, no. 8 (Oct. 2009), 16. This monthly publication (except Feb. and Aug.) delivers current events and information of interest and concern to senior Americans. (AARP, 601 E. St. N.W., Washington, D.C. 20049).
13. "Ruth Graham's Funeral Held in N.C.," CBS News, http:/www.cbsnews.com/stories/2007/06/16/national/main2939093.shtml.
14. "Ruth Graham buried at N.C. Library," U.S.A TODAY.com http://www.usatoday.com/news/nation/2007-06-17-ruth- graham-burial.
15. Becker, *Denial of Death*, 284.

Chapter VI
1. Ellen Goodman, "Denial Continues to Drive High End-of-Life Costs," *The Tennessean*, 21A, May 10, 2009. Ellen Goodman is a columnist for the Boston Globe. e-mail: ellengoodman@globe.com.
2. "Who Will Play God?" Medicine: Question. TIME, Apr. 09, 1984. http:/www.time.com/time/magazine/article/0,9171,952398,00.html, Monday.
3. Rolston, *Science and Religion*, 135-36.
4. "Gov. Lamm Asserts, Elderly, If Very Ill, Have a Duty to Die," *The New York Times*, (Document View—ProQuest), http://proquest.umi.com/pqdweb.
5. Cassell, *The Healer's Art*, 205.
6. Ibid., 209
7. Bedell, et al, "Survival after Cardio-Pulmonary Resuscitation in the Hospital *New England Journal of Medicine* 309, no. 10, (Sept. 8, 1983): 569.

8. Charlson, et al., "Resuscitation: How Do We Decide?" *Journal of American Medical Association* 255, no. 10 (March 14, 1986): 1316.
9. "Futile Care," Council On Ethical and Judicial Affairs, *American Medical Association Current Opinions*, 2004-2005, Item 2,035: 13.
10. Lisa Green, "Feeding Tubes Snake Through Medical History," TampaBay.com, http://www.sptimes.com/2005/03/news_pf/Tampabay/Feeding_tube
11. Angela Morrow, R.N., "Artificial Nutrition and Hydration: Feeding Tubes and IVs at the End-of-Life," About.com. Palliative Care, (http://dying.about.com/od/lifesupport/a/artificialfeed.htm). Updated March 14, 2011.
12. Howard Brody, et al, "Withdrawing Intensive Life-Sustaining Treatment," *New England Journal of Medicine* 336, no. 9 (Feb. 27, 1993).

Chapter VII
1. David Randolph Smith, "Legal Issues Leading to the Notion of Neo-Cortical Death," *Death: Beyond Whole-Brain Criteria,* ed. Richard L. Zaner (Dordrecht/Boston/London: Kluwer Academic Publishers, 1988), 134.
2. "The Doctors Trial," U.S. Holocaust Memorial Museum, Documents come from the official record: Trials of War Criminals before the Nuremburg Military Tribunals under Control Council Law No.10. Nuremburg, October 1946-April 1949, (Online), Exhibitions: Washington D.C. : U. S. G.P. O, 1949-1953.
3. Ibid, Nuremburg Code excerpts.
4. "Ethical and Religious Directives for Catholic Health Services," National Conference of Catholic Bishops, United States Catholic Conference, Publication No. 029-X (Washington, D.C.: 1995), Introduction, 25.
5. Ibid., Directive 62, 23.
6. "The Nature and Value of Human Life," Report of the Council on Theology and Culture, approved by the 121st. General Assembly of the Presbyterian Church, U.S. (Part I Journal, with Directory and Appendix, May 20-27, Houston, Texas), Appendix, Part II, p.290.

7. Daniel Callahan, "Sanctity of Life Seduced" A Symposium on Medical Ethics, Callahan, Meilaender, Whitbeck, Smith, Lysaught, May, Cassel, (Online, Issue Archive, First Things) April 1994.
8. Edmund D. Pelligrino, *Humanism and the Physician* (Knoxville: The University of Tennessee Press, 1979), 3-4.
9. Carol McCoy, J.D., Vanderbilt School of Law, 1973. Elected to the Bench, Chancery Court of Middle Tennessee, 1996. Professional and social friend of this author, who shared data from her file accumulated when she was appointed guardian ad litem representing Mary Northern.
10. James E. Drane, "The Many Faces of Competency" *The Hastings Center Report*, 15, no. 2 (April, 1985): 17.
11. Ibid.

Part Two

1. Richard M. Zaner, *Death: Beyond Whole-Brain Criteria*, (Dordrecht/Boston/London: Kluwer Academic Publishers, 1988), preface, viii-ix.

Chapter VIII
1. Data from author's clinical involvement over 18 year period—conversations with physicians and general information from a variety of sources within that time frame. See also Wikipedia, The Free Encyclopedia for information on the history, timeline, and use of Encephalography.
2. Sherwin B. Nuland, *How We Die: Reflections on Life's Final Chapter* (New York: First Vintage Books Edition, A Division of Random House, 1995), Intro. xviii.
3. Charles E. Curran, *Politics, Medicine, and Christian Ethics: A Dialogue with Paul Ramsey* (Philadelphia: Fortress Press, 1973), 148.

Chapter IX
1. Cerebral Hypoxia Information Page, National Institute of Neurological Disorders and Stroke, http://www.ninds.nih.gov/disorders/anoxia/anoxia.htm.
2. Medicolegal Neurology: Special Issues, http://meilhu.com/view/600213562.html.
3. Ibid.

4. "Justice delayed is justice denied," Wickipedia. Also, see Justice Delayed is Justice Denied/Facebook: http:/www.facebook.com.
5. See Zaner, *Death: Beyond Whole-Brain Criteria.*
6. David M. Greer, Panayiotis Varelas, Shamael Haque, Eelco F. Wijdicks, "Lack of Uniformity in Hospital Brain Death Guidelines in Renowned U.S. Medical Institutions," *Annals of. Neurology*, 62, Issue S11, (October 2007): 579-80.
7. See Zaner, *Death Beyond Whole-Brain Criteria,* essence of entire book.
8. The Multi-Society Task Force on PVS, "Medical Aspects of the Persistent Vegetative State," *New England Journal of Medicine* 330, no. 21 (First of two parts, May 26, 1944); 330, no. 22 (Second of two parts, June 2, 1994).
9. MSTP, Jeanette and Plum, *NEJM*, (May 26, 1944): 1499.
10. Ibid., 1503.
11. Roland Pucetti, in Zaner, *Death Beyond Whole-Brain Criteria,* 87.
12. Ibid., essence of entire book.
13. MSTP, *NEJM* (June 2, 1944), 1575.
14. Joseph and Julia Quinlan, with Phyllis Battelle, *Karen Ann: The Quinlans Tell Their Story* (New York: A Bantam Book, by arr. with Doubleday, 1977), 12.
15. In RE Quinlan, 70 N. J. 10 (1976) 355 A.2d 647, (Online).
16. National Conference of Catholic Bishops, "Ethical and Religious Directives for Catholic Health Services," no. 029-X, Item no. 57.
17. Quinlan, *Karen Ann*, 108.
18. Ibid., 109.
19. Philip Hirsch, "Applying the Principles of Nuremberg in the International Court," *Washington University Studies Law Review* 6 (2007): 501-7. See also: Nuremberg Trials 60th Anniversary, *Dimensions, A Journal of Holocaust Studies* 19 (Fall 2006), http://www.adl.org/braun/dimensions_toc.asp.
20. Cruzan v. Director of Missouri Department of Health, 497 (U.S. Supreme Court, 261 1990) June 25.
21. Quinlan, *Karen Ann*, 15-125.
22. Ibid., 142-43.
23. Ibid. IN RE QUINLAN, 70 N.J. 10 355 A.2d. 647. (N.J. Supreme Court 1976)

24. E. Esposito, 1941-1978, a reference in an article by Robert Rakestraw, Jr., *Journal of Evangelistic Theological Society JETS* 35/3, (September 1992): 389-405, ref. no.9.
25. In RE Quinlan.
26. Daniel Dilling, *Virtual Mentor* 9, no. 5 (Online) (May 2007): 359-61.
27. "Medical Aspects of Persistent Vegetative State," *New England Journal*: 1578.
28. Daniel C. Maguire, *The Moral Revolution: A Christian Humanist Vision,* (San Francisco: Harper and Row, 1986), 172. See also Catholic Moral Theologian Charles E. Curran, *Politics, Medicine, and Christian Ethics*, (Philadelphia: Fortress Press, 1973), 152-63.
29. John Lachs, "The Element of Choice in Criteria of Death," in Zaner, *Death Beyond Whole-Brain Criteria*, 251.
30. Ibid.
31. President's Commission, Whole-Brain Definition of Death, Part Two, p. 106, in this manuscript.
32. Zaner, *Death Beyond Whole-Brain Criteria*, 3.
33. Edward T. Bartlett.Ph. D. and Stuart J. Youngner, "Human Death and Destruction of Neocortex," in Zaner, *Death Beyond Whole-Brain Criteria*, 211.
34. Robert Veatch, "Whole-Brain, Neocortical, and Higher Brain," in Zaner, *Death Beyond Whole-Brain Criteria*, 173.
35. Ibid., 184-85.
36. Ibid., 182.
37. "Nature and Value of Human Life," Minutes of the 121st General Assembly, Part I, Journal. May 20-27, Houston, TX, 1981, p. 288.
38. Lachs, "The Elements of Choice," 251.
39. Martin Pernick, "Back from the Grave; Recurring Controversies over Defining and Diagnosing Death in History," in Zaner, *Death Beyond Whole-Brain Criteria*, 17.
40. Ibid., 20.
41. Ibid. 61.
42. Maguire, *The Moral Revolution*, 172.
43. Nuland, *How We Die*, 264.

44. Robert Rakestraw, "The Persistent Vegetative State and the Withdrawal of Nutrition," *Journal Evangelical Theological Journal, JETS*, 35/3 (September, 1992): 389-405.
45. David Randolph Smith, "Legal Issues Leading to the Notion of Neocortical Death," in Zaner, *Death Beyond Whole-Brain Criteria,* 128.
46. Ibid., 129.
47. Lachs, "Element of Choice," 251.
48. Mary Moore, (see chapter II, this manuscript).

Chapter X
1. Cruzan v Harmon 760 S.W. 2d. 408, 417 (MO, 1985)
2. Ibid.
3. Ibid.
4. George Annas, "Legal Issues in Medicine," *New England Journal of Medicine* 352, no. 16 (April 21, 2005): 1710.
5. Ibid., 1711.
6. Cruzan v. Harmon, 700 SW 2D 408, 416-417,
7. Cruzan v. Director Missouri Department of Health 497 U.S.261 (1990).
8. Annas, "Legal Issues," 1711.
9. Bruce White, et al, "What Does Cruzan Mean to the Practicing Physician?" *Archives of Internal Medicine* 151 (May 1991): 925-28.
10. CSA Home Page, Society of Certified Senior Advisors, Providing the Premier Educational Credentials for Professionals Serving Seniors, www.twitter.com/societycsa...
11. Union Pacific Railroad v Botsfod 141 U.S. 250, 251, (1891).
12. Mohr v Williams, 95 Minn. 261, 104, N.W. 12, 1905.
13. Schloendorff v Society of New York Hospitals, 211, N.Y., 129-30 105N.E. 92, 90 (1914).
14. Steven Entelt, ed. "Terri Schiavo Tombstone Quote Wasn't Meant to Offend Says Brother," *Life News.com*, (June 22, 2005), http://www.lifenews.com/2005/06/22/bio-1046/.
15. Timothy Quill, "Terri Schiavo—A Tragedy Compounded," *New England Journal of Medicine* 352 no.16 (April 21, 2005): 1631.

16. In RE: The Guardianship of Theresa Marie Schiavo, (Circuit Court, Pinellas County, Florida, Probate Division), File No. 90-2908GD-003.
17. In Re Guardianship of Estelle M. Browning, State of Florida, Petitioner, v. Doris F. Herbert, etc. Respondent, 568 So. 2d 4, (Supreme Court of Florida) No. 74174, Sept. 13, 1990.
18. George Annas, "Culture of Life: Politics at the Bedside—The Case of Terri Schiavo,"
New England Journal of Medicine 35216 (April 21, 205): 1710.
19. Robert Fine, "From Quinlan to Schiavo: Medical, Ethical, and Legal Issues in Severe Brain Injuries," Journal List > Proc (Bayl Univ Med Center) > v.18 (4): (2005): 303-10 (online).
20. "Terri Schiavo, Timeline, Michael appointed Guardian by court, no objection at that time from Schindlers, Terri's parents," *CBC News In Depth*, March 31, 2005, http://www.cbc.ca/news/background/schiavo.
21. In RE: The Guardianship of Theresa Marie Schiavo, Incapacitated, In the Circuit Court For Pinellas County, Florida, Probate Division, File No. 90-2908GD-003., Exhibit I. .2.
22. Ibid.
23. "Terri Schiavo Timeline," *ABC News,* Jan 6, 2006, http://abcnews.go.com/Health/Schiavo/story?id=531632&page=1.
24. Ibid.
25. Ibid.
26. "The Guardianship of Terri Schiavo Incapacitated," Exhibit I, 3
27. *Random House Webster's Dictionary*, (New York: Random House, 1995), 1305.
28. See Abstract Appeal—Conigliaro, http:L://abstract appeal.com/schiavo/infopage.html.
29. Ronald Bailey, "Terri Schiavo R.I.P: The Controversy's Aftermath One Year Later," *Reason Magazine*, http://reason.com/archives2006/03/31/terri-schiavo.rip.
30. Liza Porteus, "GOP Goes on Judicial Offensive," *Fox News*, Friday April 1, 2005. http://www.foxnews.com/story/0,2433,15095,00.html.
31. Ibid.
32. Ibid.

33. Annas, "Culture of Life," 1710.
34. In Re: "Guardianship of Terri Schiavo, Incapacitated," Exhibit 1, 6.
35. Tamara Lush, "Memorial Praises Terri," *Petersburg Times—Tampa Bay*, http://www.sptimes.com/2005/04/01/tampabay/memorial-praises-terri.html.
36. *New York Times*, October 23, 1985, http:www.nytimes.com/1985/10/23/us/judge/rejects-plea-to stop-patient-s-food.html.
37. "Refusing and Withdrawing Medical Treatment—Historical Background," http://medicine.jrank.org/pages/1449/Refusing-Withdrawing-Medical-T.
38. Joshua E. Perry, Larry Churchill, and Howard S. Kirshner, "The Terri Schiavo Case: Legal, Ethical, and Medical Perspectives," *Annals of Internal Medicine* 143 (Perspective, 2005) 143: 744-48.
39. Timothy E. Quill, "Terri Schiavo—A Tragedy Compounded," *The New England Journal of Medicine* 352, no.16, (April 21, 2005): 1630.
40. Warren E. Burger, Chief Justice, "What's Wrong with the Courts: The Chief Justice Speaks Out," *U.S, News and World Report* 69, no.8 (Aug.24, 1970): 68, 71.

Chapter XI.
1. Daniel C. Maguire, *Ethics: A Complete Method for Moral Choice,* (Minneapolis: Augsburg Fortress, 2010), 52.
2. Will Durant, *The Story of Civilization Part II, The Life of Greece,* (New York: Simon and Shuster, 1939), 254-55.
3. Howard Zinn, *A People's History of the United States*, (New York: Harper Collins, 1980), 73.
4. Ibid., 171.
5. Ibid., 73.
6. Martin Luther King, Jr., "Letter from a Birmingham Jail," *The Autobiography of Martin Luther King, Jr.,* (New York: IPM, Intellectual Properties Management, in association with Warner Books, 1988), 191-92.
7. Maguire, *Ethics*, 55.

8. Annas, "Culture of Life," 1710.
9. Charles Curran, *Politics, Medicine, and Christian Ethics*, (Philadelphia: Fortress Press, 1973), 131.
10. Annas, "Culture of Life," 1714-15.
11. William E. May, "Contraception, Gateway to the Culture of Death," Borrowed from the journal *Faith* and used by permission on the Professor May Home Page, The Catholic University of America, Washington, D.C.
 http://www.christendom-awake.org/pages/may/contraception.htm.
12. M. Gregg Bloche, "Managing Conflict at the End of Life," *New England Journal of Medicine* 352, no. 23 (June 9, 2005): 2371.
13. Aristotle, *Nicomachean Ethics*, Book I, Sec., 2, 339 (Great Books).
14. I Corinthians 14:7-8, NRSV.
15. Roland Pucetti, "Does Anyone Survive Neocortical Death?" in Zaner, *Death: Beyond Whole-Brain Criteria*, 88.
16. David Randolph Smith, "Notion of Neocortical Death," in Zaner, *Death: Beyond Whole-Brain Criteria*, 131
17. Ibid.

Part Three
Chapter XII
1. Schloendorff v. The Society of New York Hospital (105 N.E. 92) 1914.
2. Story shared through personal interview with this author by the widow of John Doe II and used with her permission, withholding names and places at her request.
3. Limited review and explication of *The Diving Bell and the Butterfly*, by Jean-Dominique Bauby, trans. Jeremy Leggett (New York: Alfred A. Knoff, 1997). Assimilated with commentary.
4. Ibid., Prologue, 3.

Chapter XIII
1. Lou.Gehrig—The Free Encyclopedia: en.wikipedia.org/wiki/lou_Gehrig.
2. Wikipedia, sec.2.1.
3. Wikipedia, sec.2.2.

4. Albert R. Jonsen, Mark Sieglar, and William J. Winslade, *Clinical Ethics*, (New York: McGraw-Hill Health Professions Division, 1998), 139.
5. Ibid.
6. Jane Doe's story was shared by her personal physician James Wilson, M.D. (deceased) in Clinical Ethics for Practitioners workshops directed by this author, as well as in newspaper articles appearing in the *Nashville Banner*, (later retrieved from Banner Archives in Nashville-Davidson County Public Library) along with court documents, Doe v. Wilson, No. 90-364—II, slip op at 1—2 (Chancery Court, Davidson County, TN, filed Feb. 12, 1990).
7. *Nashville Banner*, February 7, 1990.
8. This quote and other salient facts of the Jane Doe case were shared in several Nashville area workshops directed by this author in concert with local medical centers in 1900-1991.
9. Doe v. Wilson, Legal brief filed in Chancery Court of Chancellor C. Allen High by Attorney Schaffner, February 12, 1990.
10. Schaffner brief as argument in behalf of Plaintiff Jane Doe.
11. Statement, as part of ruling by Chancellor High.
12. Editorial in *Nashville Banner* on February 12, 1990.
13. *Nashville Banner*, February 9, 1990.
14. Nancy Gamble's story was shared by her personal physician, James Sullivan, in Clinical Ethics for Practitioners workshops directed by this author in several Nashville medical centers and in newspaper articles, as well as in court documents, Nancy Gamble v. Baptist Hospital, Filed in Nashville—Davidson County Chancery Court April 10, 1990. No. 90—1021—III, Book 56, p.737. Attorney Mary Martin Schaffner was Gamble's attorney as she was for Jane Doe in the preceding case. Dr. Sullivan is currently practicing with the Meharry Medical Group in Nashville.
15. Bill Snyder Senior Medical Writer, *Nashville Banner*, April 3, 1990.
16. Kirk Loggins, Staff Writer, *Nashville Banner*, April 4, 1990.
17. Bill Snyder, Senior Medical Writer, *Nashville Banner*, April 3, 1990.
18. "Woman Dies after Judge OK'd Respirator Removal." *Los Angeles Times*-United Press International, April 11, 1990, articles.latimes.com/1990-04-//...mn-1274-1-woman-died-today.

19. Brief file in court of Chancellor Robert Brandt, Nancy Gamble v. Baptist Hospital, April 10, 1990.
20. Rebuttal argument filed in brief of Attorney Schaffner and made part of Chancellor's judgment on April 10, 1990.
21. Bill Snyder, Senior Medical Writer, *Nashville Banner*, April 10, 1990.
22. Arguments heard and judgment rendered by Chancellor Robert Brandt, April 10, 1990.
23. Jim Molpus and Bill Snyder, *Banner* Staff Writers, *Nashville Banner*, April 11, 1990.
24. Ellen Dahnke, Staff Writer, *Nashville Banner*, April 12, 1990.
25. Daniel Maguire, *The Moral Revolution: A Christian Humanist Vision* (San Francisco: Harper and Row, 1986), 178.

Epilogue
1. Psalm 84:3, NRSV.
2. Matthew 10:29, NRSV.
3. Nuland, *How We Die*, 262.
4. Matthew 10:31, NRSV.

C. Robert Test

A writer named Robert N. Test made his extraordinary poetic legacy available to donor services, churches, funeral homes, and other helping agencies throughout the country before his death in 1994. He and his family hoped that it would inspire many to consider the donation of body parts to those desperately in need of them. I do not know of any other written statement that has so eloquently and compassionately expressed the concern of those who are dedicated to the cause of organ donation. Our appreciation is extended to him posthumously and to the surviving members of his family.

To Remember Me

The day will come when my body will lie upon a white sheet neatly tucked under four corners of a mattress located in a hospital busily occupied with the living and the dying. **At** a certain moment a doctor will determine that my brain has ceased to function and that, for all intents and purposes, my life has stopped. **When** that happens, do not attempt to instill artificial life into my body by the use of a machine. **Let** it be called the Bed of Life, and let my body be taken from it to help others lead fuller lives.

> **Give** my sight to the man who has never seen a sunrise, a baby's face or love in the eyes of a woman.
> **Give** my heart to the person whose own heart has caused nothing but endless days of pain.
> **Give** my blood to the teenager who was pulled from the wreckage of his car, so that he might live to see his grandchildren play.
> **Give** my kidneys to one who depends on a machine to exist from week to week.
> **Take** my bones, every muscle, every fiber and nerve in my body and find a way to make a crippled child walk.
> **Explore** every corner of my brain.
> **Take** my cells, if necessary, and let them grow so that, someday, a speechless boy will shout at the crack of a bat and a human being can now be identified technologically with certainty. If there is still some question, PET studies of cerebral blood flow and glucose metabolism give further confirmation of whether or not the deaf girl will hear the sound of rain against her window.
> **Burn** what is left of me and scatter the ashes to the winds to help the flowers grow.
> **If** you bury something, let it be my faults, my

weaknesses and all prejudice against my fellow man.
Give my sins to the devil.
Give my soul to God.
If, by chance, you wish to remember me, do it with
a kind deed or word to someone who needs you.
If you do all I have asked, I will live forever.

Robert N. Test

D. End-of-Life Helping Agencies

1. **"Compassionate Friends."** Their expressed mission is "To assist families toward the positive resolution of grief following the death of a child of any age and to provide information to help others be supportive." Contact Information is:
>The Compassionate Friends, Inc
>P.O. Box 3696
>Oak Brook, IL 60522-3696
>Toll-Free: 877-969-0010
>PH: 630-990-0010
>FAX: 630-990-0246

2. The nation's most comprehensive resource for "choice" in dying is a highly respected group called **"Compassion and Choices."** Contact address below:
>**Compassion and Choices**
>P.O. Box 101810
>Denver, CO 80250 – 1810
>800 – 247 – 7421 (t)
>303 – 639 – 1224 (f)

3. **Presumed Consent Foundation, Inc.**
www.presumedconsent.org
Dedicated to making organ transplantation to all who need it.

4. **Caring Connection:** A program of the National Hospice and Palliative Care
Organization—Consumer Web Site: www.caringinfo.org
Toll-free HelpLine: 1-800-658-8898

>Order paperback copies from:
>Amazon CreateSpace   or
>Electronic Edition from:
>The Kindle Store (KDP Select)

About the Author

Robert Henry Crumby is a graduate of Rhodes College, with postgraduate degrees from Presbyterian Seminaries in Richmond, Virginia and Louisville, Kentucky. He earned the professional Doctor of Ministry Degree in Social and Political Ethics at Vanderbilt University. In 1992, he redirected professionally from the active Presbyterian Ministry after 36 years of pastoral service with churches and communities in Alabama, Kentucky, and Tennessee. He was Adjunct Assistant Professor of Medical Ethics and Associate Director of the Center for Clinical and Research Ethics at Vanderbilt School of Medicine, taught Clinical Medical Ethics at Meharry Medical College, was a consultant in clinical ethics for Hospital Corporation of America, and founded centers for clinical ethics in two H.C.A. Medical Centers in Nashville, Summit and Skyline. Retiring altogether in 2003, Robert and Judith, his wife of 54 years, have 2 daughters and 1 son, along with 6 grandchildren.

Made in the USA
Charleston, SC
17 June 2013